DIABETES HEAD TO TOE

DIABETES
HEAD TO TOE

Everything You Need to Know about Diagnosis, Treatment, and Living with Diabetes

RITA R. KALYANI, MD, MHS

MARK D. CORRIERE, MD

THOMAS W. DONNER, MD

MICHAEL W. QUARTUCCIO, MD

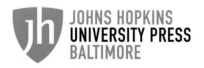
JOHNS HOPKINS
UNIVERSITY PRESS
BALTIMORE

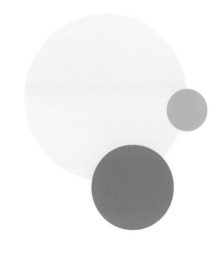

© 2018 Johns Hopkins University Press
All rights reserved. Published 2018
Printed in Canada on acid-free paper
9 8 7 6 5 4 3 2 1

Johns Hopkins University Press
2715 North Charles Street
Baltimore, Maryland 21218-4363
www.press.jhu.edu

Library of Congress Cataloging-in-Publication Data
Names: Kalyani, Rita Rastogi, author.
Title: Diabetes head to toe : everything you need to know about diagnosis, treatment, and living
   with diabetes / Rita R. Kalyani, MD, MHS, Mark D. Corriere, MD, Thomas W. Donner, MD,
   Michael W. Quartuccio, MD.
Description: Baltimore : Johns Hopkins University Press, 2018. | Series: A Johns Hopkins Press
   health book | Includes bibliographical references and index.
Identifiers: LCCN 2018000282 | ISBN 9781421426471 (hardcover : alk. paper) |
   ISBN 1421426471 (hardcover : alk. paper) | ISBN 9781421426488 (paperback : alk. paper) |
   ISBN 142142648X (paperback : alk. paper) | ISBN 9781421426495 (electronic) |
   ISBN 1421426498 (electronic)
Subjects: LCSH: Diabetes—Diagnosis—Popular works. | Diabetes—Treatment—Popular works.
Classification: LCC RA645.D5 K35 2018 | DDC 616.4/62—dc23
LC record available at https://lccn.loc.gov/2018000282

A catalog record for this book is available from the British Library.

Illustrations by Jennifer E. Fairman, MA, CMI, FAMI, and Tim Phelps, MS, FAMI
© 2018, Johns Hopkins University, Art as Applied to Medicine

Special discounts are available for bulk purchases of this book. For more information, please contact Special Sales at 410-516-6936 or specialsales@press.jhu.edu.

Johns Hopkins University Press uses environmentally friendly book materials, including recycled text paper that is composed of at least 30 percent post-consumer waste, whenever possible.

To the millions of people living with diabetes worldwide whose inspiring stories and determination give us hope. To my husband, Sachin, and my children, Shaan and Sonia, who are my constant source of wisdom, joy, and pride, and to my parents for always seeing what is possible.

—RITA R. KALYANI

To my wife, Suzy, and children—Dominic, Molly, Sam, and Tommy—for their constant support and encouragement of my career. To my dad, who was the first person to pique my interest in diabetes, and the scores of patients I have been honored to treat who have grown my interest in this field.

—MARK D. CORRIERE

To my wife, Danielle, and my children—Gabriel, Bridget, and Celia—who so enrich my life. And to my patients who have had the courage and persistence to take on this challenging disease and from whom I have learned so much.

—THOMAS W. DONNER

To my wife, Katelyn, and son, Benjamin, who have been so supportive of my career choice. To my parents, who constantly pushed me to achieve my goals. And to all my patients, who inspire me to work harder every day.

—MICHAEL W. QUARTUCCIO

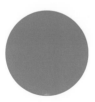

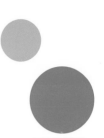

CONTENTS

PREFACE

We wrote this book for you. Chances are that you either know someone who has diabetes, are at risk of developing diabetes, or have diabetes yourself. The number of people with diabetes continues to climb dramatically, and the face of diabetes worldwide is changing rapidly. No two people with diabetes are alike. There are various types of diabetes, and some people are more likely to develop diabetes than others. An ever-increasing number of medications are available to treat this disease. While some people need insulin right away, others do not. The disease can affect many different organs in the body—from head to toe and everywhere in between. Not everyone with diabetes develops the same complications or medical conditions.

The information in these pages represents the best of what we know to date. We are health professionals who have not only spent many years specializing in the comprehensive care of people with diabetes but who have also established clinical guidelines for how all health professionals should care for people with diabetes. We treat people with diabetes both in the community and in university-based centers. We are hopeful that patients, family members, teachers, physicians, nurses, dietitians, pharmacists, specialists, and anyone else who cares about the health of a person with diabetes will benefit from this book.

Diabetes is a chronic illness that relies heavily on a person's ability to self-manage his or her disease. Yet during a routine clinic visit, health care providers may be limited (for a variety of reasons) in their ability to relay the critical information that people with diabetes need to optimally manage their disease at home. Many complications of diabetes are preventable. By reading this book, we hope that people with diabetes will be better equipped to recognize early warning signs so that the appropriate measures can be taken. This will help to avoid difficulties in the future. The goal is attainable, but it starts with you.

In this book, we provide up-to-date information written in simple, easy-to-grasp sections. We emphasize the key facts that we would want any person who has diabetes (or who is interested in diabetes) to know—as if we were sitting face-to-face with you right now. The more than 130 topics in this book cover the different ways in which diabetes can affect a person from a personal, family, societal, and legal perspective. This book goes beyond describing the "traditional" small blood vessel complications (eye disease, kidney disease, and nerve disease) and large blood vessel complications (heart disease, stroke, and peripheral artery disease) of diabetes that, while undoubtedly important, do not fully capture how diabetes can affect the day-to-day life of someone living with the disease. The wide breadth of topics and easy accessibility of the content have the goal of empowering you with the critical knowledge you need to confidently self-manage diabetes at home and to facilitate informed discussions with your health care team.

Each topic begins with a short introduction that defines the medical conditions in plain everyday language. The technical medical terms are also included to familiarize you with them. The next section for each topic is titled "What You Need to Know" and outlines the important facts for each topic. The last section of each topic, titled "What Does It All Mean?" distills in a few sentences or bullet points the key items for each topic and the action steps you can take today. While the sections for each topic are intended to be read in the order written, you may decide to read the last section first to grasp the key points from the beginning. The topics are not meant to be extensive in length but instead, may trigger you to seek more information about a specific area of interest. You will notice that "health care provider" is used intentionally throughout the book in order to include physicians, nurse practitioners, dietitians, pharmacists, podiatrists, and all the other specialists who may be involved in the comprehensive care of people with diabetes.

The book is arranged in 12 chapters:

- Chapter 1 gives a quick introduction to diabetes, along with key facts about its rising global and economic impact. It includes a brief description of the landmark studies that form the basis for our current thinking on how to manage and treat diabetes today.
- Chapter 2 covers how the two main types of diabetes (type 1 and type 2) and

prediabetes are diagnosed, presents common risk factors for the disease, and briefly describes other forms of diabetes (such as steroid-induced diabetes).

○ Chapter 3 goes over the general aspects of blood glucose monitoring, recognizing the symptoms of high blood glucose (*hyperglycemia*) emergencies and low blood glucose (*hypoglycemia*) and how to treat it; the importance of routine preventive care and vaccinations; and societal and legal issues, such as driving if you have diabetes and employment discrimination.

○ Chapter 4 discusses diabetes management in special populations, such as children or older adults, and among people from different cultures or racial groups. It also presents information on how diabetes may be managed differently in the hospital and after pancreatic surgery.

○ Chapter 5 focuses on the importance of lifestyle and behavioral changes— the foundation of care for all people with diabetes—and discusses healthy nutrition, physical exercise, diabetes self-management education, and ways to overcome common fears and other obstacles to good health.

○ Chapter 6 highlights the role of managing obesity and bariatric surgery, particularly in people with type 2 diabetes.

○ Chapter 7 forms the backbone of this book and goes through, in sequence from head to toe, the many different body organs that diabetes can affect. You may want to read this part from beginning to end, or you may prefer to turn to specific sections that address the areas of relevance or concern to you right now. You may be surprised to find that diabetes can affect so many parts of the body, such as the gums (*periodontal disease*), liver (*nonalcoholic fatty liver disease*), and bones (*osteoporosis*), for instance, or that diabetes is linked to a higher risk for depression, hearing loss, and certain cancers. Diabetes can also affect both men's and women's sexual function. In particular, diabetes needs to be managed especially carefully just before and during pregnancy, and all pregnant women should be screened for diabetes, which can develop for the first time during pregnancy (called *gestational diabetes*).

○ Chapter 8 provides an overview of treatments for type 1 and type 2 diabetes (which may overlap with treatments for gestational diabetes and other forms of diabetes as well).

○ Chapter 9 then dives into the rising number of medications available for people with diabetes and the choices for treatment on the market, including pills, injected and inhaled insulin, and medications that are also injected but are not insulin. Recognizing the use of complementary and alternative treatments by many people with diabetes, information is also given on this topic.

- Chapter 10 goes over commonly prescribed medications to treat high blood pressure (*hypertension*), address cholesterol abnormalities (*dyslipidemia*), and prevent heart disease and stroke (*cardiovascular disease*) in people with diabetes.
- Chapter 11 highlights the current technologies available to help monitor blood glucose levels or deliver insulin and their increasing use in the treatment of people with diabetes.
- Chapter 12 ends with information on cutting-edge and future treatments for diabetes, including pancreas and islet transplantation, and the quest to develop an artificial pancreas. We are getting closer but are still not quite there.

Our knowledge of diabetes—and how best to treat the disease—is evolving rapidly. There are exciting developments sure to come that will make the daily management even easier for people living with diabetes in the future. We have strived in this book to relay to you the best of what we, as health professionals, know to date in a format that is quickly and easily accessible. Throughout the book, we include information on the different ways that diabetes can affect people from head to toe so that you can understand its wide-ranging impact. Most importantly, we emphasize the things you can do to prevent these complications—small but incrementally important steps that can add up to good health in the long run. In the process, you may find out something new about diabetes that you didn't know. If at any point while reading this book you say to yourself, "No one told me that could happen with diabetes," then this book has achieved its purpose. And taking that critical jump to understanding what you don't know—and what you can do now for your well-being—is what will ensure that you live a long, healthy life with diabetes. Your guide awaits in the pages ahead.

ACKNOWLEDGMENTS

We thank the patients and colleagues, representing the different professions and specialties involved in the comprehensive care of people with diabetes, who reviewed selected topics in this book, including Mohammed Al-Sofiani, MBBS, MSc; Pamela Allweiss, MD, MPH; Nicholas Argento, MD; Nisha Aurora, MD; Holly Bashura, CRNP, CDE; Scott Blackman, MD, PhD; David Cooke, MD; Deidra C. Crews, MD, MSc; Stacy Elder Dalpoas, PharmD; Meg Gerstenblith, MD; Sheldon Gottlieb, MD; Erica Hall, CRNP, CDE; Sachin Kalyani, MD; Paul Ladenson, MD; Clare Lee, MD, MHS; Frank Lin, MD, PhD; Megan Lobus, MS, RD, CDE; Rebecca Manno, MD, MHS; Christine McKinney, MS, RD, LDN, CDE; Anne Monroe, MD, MPH; Joshua Neumiller, PharmD, CDE; Anna Norton, MS; Damani Pigott, MD, PhD; Brian Pinto, PharmD, MBA; Susan Renda, DNP, CDE; Lee Sanders, DPM; Erica Schuyler, MD; Maureen Seel, RD, LDN, CDE; Steven Tsamoutalis, BS; and Swaytha Yalamanchi, MD.

We particularly thank William H. Herman, MD, MPH, for his helpful and comprehensive review of the book.

We appreciate the support of our colleagues in the Johns Hopkins Division of Endocrinology, Diabetes, and Metabolism and Thomas N. Mitchell, BA, for his assistance.

We acknowledge the remarkable contributions of Jennifer E. Fairman, MA, CMI, FAMI, and Tim Phelps, MS, FAMI, for the illustrations in this book.

We are incredibly grateful for the assistance and support of our editors at Johns Hopkins University Press, especially Joe Rusko, and Jacqueline C. Wehmueller, MA, whose input was crucial at all stages of writing our book. We also thank Juliana McCarthy, MA, our managing editor, and Wendy Lawrence, our copy editor, for their tremendous assistance. We would like to acknowledge the editorial services of Ann Griswold.

We specifically acknowledge our families for their patience and support as we worked on this book.

Finally, we acknowledge the many patients and their families who have helped us understand what they want to know about caring for themselves or loved ones with diabetes and who have encouraged us to write this book.

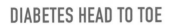

DIABETES HEAD TO TOE

Chapter 1

A QUICK OVERVIEW OF DIABETES

Introduction to Diabetes

Diabetes is a disease in which there is too much glucose ("sugar") in the blood. People with diabetes cannot maintain healthy levels of blood glucose unless they carefully adjust their lifestyles and, in most cases, take medications. Although everyone may occasionally experience bouts of high blood glucose, people with diabetes experience this problem more severely and frequently unless appropriately treated. Abnormally high blood glucose levels that persist over time can lead to a number of serious health complications.

▶ WHAT YOU NEED TO KNOW

What Causes Blood Glucose to Rise

A small fraction of people with diabetes (about 5%) have *type 1 diabetes*. They lose the ability to make *insulin*—a hormone the pancreas produces to help the body process carbohydrates from meals—because of the destruction of pancreatic tissue.

Most people with diabetes (about 90% to 95%) have *type 2 diabetes*. Although these people can produce insulin early in the disease, the amount is not sufficient to effectively lower blood glucose levels. In other words, the body is *resistant* to the effects of insulin. The pancreas tries to overcome this by manufacturing more insulin. After a while the pancreas can no longer produce enough insulin and diabetes develops (see "Diagnosing Diabetes" on page 11).

Gestational diabetes is a type of diabetes diagnosed in women during pregnancy. Less common types of diabetes, such as those related to defects in specific genes, also exist (for an example, see "Maturity-Onset Diabetes of the Young" on page 22).

Many organs in the body contribute to high blood glucose levels in people with diabetes. The pancreas, the only place that produces insulin, is impaired in all types of diabetes. In type 1 diabetes, the pancreas is destroyed and cannot make any insulin. In other types, the pancreas is strained and unable to produce enough insulin to meet the body's needs and keep high blood glucose levels in check.

Insulin usually helps glucose enter cells in the skeletal muscle and fat tissue and promotes the storage of glucose as glycogen in the liver. But in type 2 diabetes, these organs are resistant to insulin's effects, and glucose stays in the blood longer. The gastrointestinal tract produces hormones called *incretins* (such as GLP-1) after eating, which then stimulate the pancreas to manufacture more insulin. In persons with diabetes, these hormones may not work as well. The kidneys also usually allow a small amount of glucose to be lost in the urine when blood glucose levels run high; people with type 2 diabetes do not lose as much glucose in the urine, so blood levels stay higher. Lastly, the brain has multiple roles in stimulating the appetite in response to hormones, such as the incretins, and may be affected in people with type 2 diabetes (figure 1.1).

What Common Health Problems Occur in People with Diabetes?

Persons with any type of diabetes are at risk of developing complications. Generally, these problems fall into one of two categories:

1 *Acute* problems arise quickly and improve with prompt treatment. For example, eating too many carbohydrates or forgetting to take a medication can lead to high blood glucose levels in people with diabetes. This can cause blurry vision, fatigue, thirst, and frequent urination until treatment is given.

2 *Chronic* problems develop over many years, when blood glucose levels remain persistently high for a long period of time. They are difficult to reverse. For example, people whose diabetes has been poorly managed for many years often sustain damage to blood vessels, both big and small, throughout the body—frequently described as the "traditional" complications of diabetes. Specifically, people with diabetes are twice as likely as others to develop heart disease, stroke, and disease in the peripheral blood vessels. They are also at risk for developing complications in the eyes, nerves, and kidneys.

People with diabetes are more likely to develop diseases in other organ systems, including liver disease, bone disease (*osteoporosis*), or sexual dysfunction.

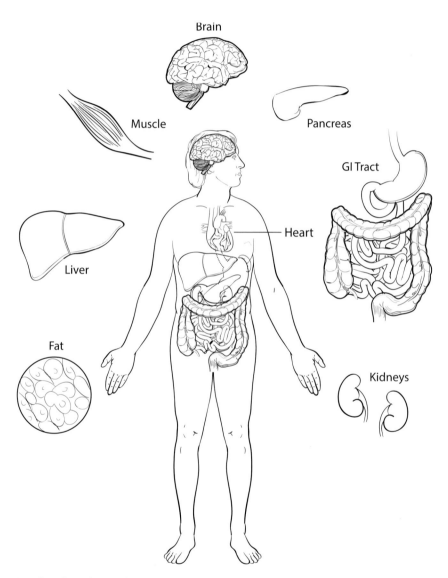

1.1 Though insulin is only produced in the pancreas, many organs in the body are involved in regulating blood glucose levels. © 2018, Johns Hopkins University, Art as Applied to Medicine

These medical conditions related to diabetes are important to identify since they can affect the daily self-management of diabetes and a person's overall quality of life and life span.

How Is Diabetes Treated?

Multiple options are available for treating diabetes. Persons with type 1 diabetes must always take insulin to control their blood glucose. Some people with type 2 diabetes can control their blood glucose by monitoring their diet and increasing their physical activity, but most require oral or injectable medications (that are not insulin) and eventually, may need to take insulin.

WHAT DOES IT ALL MEAN?

- Diabetes is a serious disease that can lead to a number of health complications. A wide range of medical conditions are more common in people with diabetes.
- With proper self-care and treatment, diabetes can be well managed—and many of its complications prevented.
- Eat healthy and exercise often. If you smoke, stop. Work with your health care providers to manage your blood pressure and cholesterol.
- Diabetes is a growing problem in the United States and around the world. This disease is expensive to treat and can lead to early death if undiagnosed or left untreated.

The Global Burden of Diabetes

In recent decades the number of people living with diabetes worldwide has surged dramatically. Diabetes is a disease that affects people of diverse backgrounds. The global burden of diabetes refers to the impact of the disease on society as measured by complication rates, early death, financial cost, and other indicators.

▶ WHAT YOU NEED TO KNOW

Ten Key Facts

1 Between 1980 and 2014, the number of adults with diabetes worldwide quadrupled. More than 400 million people in the world (about 1 in 11) have diabetes. Of great concern is the fact that the rate of people with prediabetes (when blood glucose levels are higher than normal but not high enough to be called diabetes) continues to rise.

2 More than 1 million children and adolescents in the world have type 1 diabetes. Type 2 diabetes in children is also increasing rapidly, especially among youth from minority racial and ethnic groups.

3 In the United States in 2015, about 30 million (or 9.4% of the population) had diabetes, and 84 million adults had prediabetes. About one-quarter of U.S. adults with type 2 diabetes and more than three-quarters of those with prediabetes do not realize they have the condition.

4 African Americans, Hispanics, Native Americans, and Asian Americans are much more likely to develop type 2 diabetes.

5 Diabetes is quickly becoming a problem among older adults. About three-quarters of U.S. adults aged 65 years and older have diabetes or prediabetes.

6 Type 2 diabetes is expensive to treat. Persons with diabetes spend over twice as much on medical treatment as those without diabetes. The United States spends more than $300 billion a year treating patients with diabetes—more money than any other nation in the world. One of every four U.S. health care dollars goes to caring for people with diabetes.

7 Cardiovascular disease (including heart disease and stroke) is the primary cause of death in diabetes. Diabetes results in more deaths than AIDS and breast cancer combined and is one of the top 10 leading causes of death in the United States.

8 Diabetes is a worldwide problem, with the greatest number of people with diabetes living in China and India. Diabetes is also a growing problem in the Middle East, where a particularly high percentage of the population has diabetes.

9 As the number of people with diabetes continues to rise globally, the burden of complications related to diabetes will also increase, especially in low- and middle-income countries.

10 Diabetes is a leading cause of blindness, kidney disease, nerve damage, and amputation. Almost half of all new cases of kidney failure occur in people with diabetes. But with good blood glucose levels and self-management, many of these complications are preventable.

WHAT DOES IT ALL MEAN?

- Many persons with type 2 diabetes (and prediabetes) are undiagnosed, presenting a challenge to reducing this disease's burden on society.

- Diabetes is costly, with expenses that are potentially avoidable with proper treatment.
- Ethnic minorities are more likely to develop diabetes, and the rates of diabetes are rising rapidly, especially in low- and middle-income countries, making diabetes a global concern.
- Programs that increase the awareness of diabetes and its complications and provide resources for treatment are vital to improving population health.

Landmark Studies in Diabetes Care

In the past 25 years, several large research studies in persons with prediabetes and diabetes have led to a great deal of important, scientifically supported information. These studies have shown how to effectively prevent diabetes and its complications and how, in some persons with diabetes at high risk for cardiovascular disease, less intensive targets for blood glucose control may be safer.

Some of the most important findings in diabetes prevention and blood glucose control are summarized here. This list does not include all studies to date but reveals those that have arguably had the greatest impact on the current management of diabetes.

▶ WHAT YOU NEED TO KNOW

Studies on the Prevention of Diabetes

Da Qing Study Chinese researchers randomly assigned 577 men and women with prediabetes to different diabetes prevention treatments from 1986 to 1992. They found that regular exercise and a healthy diet can reduce the risk of developing type 2 diabetes. People who modified their diet over an average period of 6 years had a 31% lower risk of diabetes, while those who adopted an exercise regimen had a 46% lower risk. People who embraced both diet and exercise lifestyle changes had a 42% lower risk compared to those who continued their usual diet and exercise patterns. The benefits of these lifestyle changes for preventing diabetes persisted up to 14 years later.

The Finnish Diabetes Prevention Study In this study, Finnish researchers randomly assigned 522 overweight middle-aged adults with prediabetes to receive intensive dietary counseling along with regular exercise or continue their usual diet and exercise patterns from 1993 to 1998. After an average of 3 years, 11% of people in the intensive lifestyle group developed diabetes compared to 23% in the usual care group, representing a 58% reduction in the risk of diabetes. The benefits of these intensive lifestyle changes for preventing diabetes persisted up to 9 years later.

Diabetes Prevention Program (DPP) In this key U.S. study from 1996 to 2001 of 3,234 overweight middle-aged adults with prediabetes, each person was randomly assigned to either an intensive lifestyle change, metformin, or placebo pills. Over an average of 3 years, the study found that those assigned to the intensive lifestyle change, which included healthier eating (based on individualized daily calorie and dietary fat goals), regular exercise (a total of 150 minutes of moderate physical activity every week, such as brisk walking for 30 minutes every day, 5 days a week), and a goal of 7% weight loss (for example, in a person who weighs 200 pounds, this would correspond to a 14-pound weight loss), reduced their risk of developing type 2 diabetes by 58% compared to the placebo group. In comparison, metformin treatment reduced the onset of diabetes by 31%. The lifestyle changes were particularly effective in persons 60 years and over and lessened this age group's risk of diabetes by 71%. The benefits of reducing the development of type 2 diabetes persisted for up to 15 years for both the lifestyle and metformin groups, supporting the importance of type 2 diabetes prevention.

Studies of type 1 diabetes have found no evidence that the early use of injected or oral insulin in people at high risk for the disease can prevent or delay its onset. Research on treatments that alter the immune system (*immune-modulating therapies*) to delay or prevent the development of type 1 diabetes is ongoing.

Studies on the Optimal Blood Glucose Targets for People with Diabetes

Diabetes Control and Complications Trial/Epidemiology of Diabetes Interventions and Complications (DCCT/EDIC) Study In this important U.S. study, 1,441 people with type 1 diabetes were randomly assigned to either an intensive or a conventional diabetes treatment from 1983 to 1993. Researchers found that damage to the retina, known as *diabetic retinopathy*, was dramatically reduced by maintaining an average A1C of 7% or 53 millimoles per mole (mmol/mol) in the intensively treated group compared to an average A1C of 9% or 75 mmol/mol in the conventionally treated group over an average 6.5-year period. Intensive blood glucose control also reduced the incidence of kidney disease and nerve damage, resulting in a 35% to 75% decrease in developing these types of small blood vessel (*microvascular*) complications during this period. However, people with tightly controlled blood glucose levels were also more likely to experience low blood glucose levels (*hypoglycemia*).

A long-term follow-up found that participants continued to benefit after the trial ended despite a slight deterioration in the glucose control of the intensively treated group and an improvement in the glucose control of the conventionally treated group. After 17 years, the group who had initially received intensive treatment had a 42% reduction in major cardiovascular events (nonfatal heart attack, stroke, or cardiovascular death) and at 30 years, modestly decreased rates of death from any cause. This all appears to be related to the 6.5 years of better glucose control during the early treatment phase of the study, suggesting that such management early in type 1 diabetes can delay or prevent cardiovascular disease.

UK Prospective Diabetes Study (UKPDS) In this hallmark study from 1977 to 1997, 5,102 people with newly diagnosed type 2 diabetes in the United Kingdom were randomly assigned to intensive therapy, leading to tighter blood glucose control (average A1C of 7% or 53 mmol/mol), compared to a group receiving conventional therapy (average A1C of 7.9% or 63 mmol/mol). Over a 10-year period, the risk of diabetes microvascular complications, including eye, kidney, and nerve disease, decreased by about 25%.

A follow-up study of these patients over another 10 years after the trial ended found a lower risk of cardiovascular disease and death from any cause in the previously more intensively treated group.

Action to Control Cardiovascular Risk in Diabetes (ACCORD) Researchers in North America randomly assigned 10,251 older people (average age 62 years) with type 2 diabetes and a high risk or history of cardiovascular disease to a very intensive versus standard therapy group from 2001 to 2008. They found that trying to achieve an A1C of less than 6% (42 mmol/mol) in the intensive therapy group (compared to an A1C between 7% to 7.9% [53 to 63 mmol/mol] in the standard therapy group) increased the risk of death from any cause after just an average of 3.5 years. This was the first major trial to suggest that a very intensive treatment regimen in people with type 2 diabetes at high risk for heart disease might lead to harm. However, the overall risk of developing *albuminuria* (an early sign of kidney disease) was much less among those very intensively treated.

Action in Diabetes and Vascular Disease: Preterax and Diamicron Modified Release Controlled Evaluation (ADVANCE) Another study of 11,140 older adults with type 2 diabetes in multiple countries investigated the benefits of intensive glucose control over 5 years from 2001 to 2007. The intensive control group (average A1C of 6.5% or 48 mmol/mol) versus the standard therapy group (average A1C of 7.3% or 56 mmol/mol) had lower overall rates of diabetic complications, primarily due to a 21% reduction in kidney disease. However, cardiovascular disease (such as heart attack or stroke) and death were not dramatically reduced, even in a long-term follow-up study after the trial was completed.

Veterans Affairs Diabetes Trial (VADT) This trial involving 1,791 older U.S. male military veterans with type 2 diabetes studied the effects of intensive glucose control over an average of 6 years from 2000 to 2008. The trial showed lower rates in the progression of diabetic kidney disease in the intensive treatment group (average A1C of 6.9% or 52 mmol/mol) compared to the standard treatment group (average A1C of 8.4% or 68 mmol/mol). Though not found during the initial trial, a follow-up study demonstrated lower rates of a first cardiovascular event in the intensive treatment group but no difference in survival.

Normoglycemia in Intensive Care Evaluation—Survival Using Glucose Algorithm Regulation (NICE—SUGAR) Trial This 2004 to 2008 study looked at 6,104 people in multiple countries with type 2 diabetes who were admitted to an intensive care unit and expected to stay at least 3 days. The study investigated the effects of tight glucose control, with a goal of 81 to 108 milligrams per deciliter (mg/dL) or 4.4 to 10 millimoles per liter (mmol/L), versus conventional therapy, with a goal of less than 180 mg/dL or 10 mmol/L, during hospitalization. Surprisingly, it found that intensive glucose control in the intensive care hospital setting led to *more* deaths than conventional approaches.

WHAT DOES IT ALL MEAN?

- Lifestyle changes (most importantly weight loss and exercise) and certain medications (such as metformin) can delay or prevent the progression from prediabetes to type 2 diabetes.
- Type 1 diabetes is more difficult to prevent. Some studies are exploring the use of drugs that suppress the immune system that may at least slow this condition, though side effects can develop from such treatments.
- Tightly managing blood glucose levels (A1C of less than 7% or 53 mmol/mol) after a diagnosis of type 1 or type 2 diabetes leads to lower rates of microvascular complications (such as eye, kidney, and nerve damage) and, in long-term follow-up, cardiovascular events (such as heart disease or stroke) and likely death.
- Vision loss and kidney damage in particular can be prevented by maintaining near-normal A1C levels over many years.
- Some studies, however, suggest that very tightly managing A1C levels to less than 6% or 6.5% (42 to 48 mmol/mol) may actually do harm to certain people with type 2 diabetes and cardiovascular disease, particularly those who have had diabetes for a long time.

- Each person with diabetes likely needs an individualized A1C goal that depends on age, medical history, and other factors.
- Aggressive glucose goals during hospital stays may lead to dangerously low glucose levels (hypoglycemia) and higher rates of death. A target that keeps glucose levels between 140 to 180 mg/dL (7.8 to 10 mmol/L) in the hospital appears to lead to better outcomes.

Chapter 2

DIAGNOSIS, SCREENING, AND TYPES OF DIABETES

Diagnosing Diabetes

How do you find out if you have diabetes? A number of different tests can be used to diagnose diabetes. All these tests directly or indirectly measure glucose levels in the blood. Sometimes people have symptoms of diabetes but other times high blood glucose levels may be found unexpectedly on a routine blood test. There may also be more specific tests performed to classify the type of diabetes (that is, autoantibody tests for type 1 diabetes; see "Testing for Autoantibodies" on page 193).

▶ WHAT YOU NEED TO KNOW

According to the American Diabetes Association, persons are diagnosed with diabetes if *any* of the following tests are abnormal:

- **Fasting blood glucose** A blood glucose level of 126 milligrams per deciliter (mg/dL) or 7.0 millimoles per liter (mmol/L) or higher after fasting (without any food or drink except water for at least 8 hours) is diagnostic of diabetes (levels of 100 to 125 mg/dL or 5.6 to 6.9 mmol/L suggest prediabetes).
- **Random blood glucose** A blood glucose level of 200 mg/dL (11.1 mmol/L) or higher at any time of day, including after eating, when the person feels symptoms of high blood glucose, such as thirstiness or blurry vision, is diagnostic of diabetes (levels between 140 to 199 mg/dL or 7.8 to 11.0 mmol/L suggest prediabetes).
- **Oral glucose tolerance test (OGTT)** A blood glucose level of 200 mg/dL (11.1 mmol/L) or higher 2 hours after consuming a 75-gram carbohydrate-contain-

ing sugary drink as part of the test is diagnostic of diabetes (levels between 140 to 199 mg/dL or 7.8 to 11.0 mmol/L suggest prediabetes).

- **Hemoglobin A1C** A hemoglobin A1C level of 6.5% or 48 millimoles per mole (mmol/mol) or higher is diagnostic of diabetes (levels between 5.7% to 6.4% or 39 to 47 mmol/mol suggest prediabetes). This test can be done at any time of day and reflects the average blood glucose levels over the past 3 months (see "Hemoglobin A1C Testing" on page 33).

The abnormal test should be repeated on a separate day to ensure there was no laboratory error and that the blood glucose levels are definitely high. Sometimes a person can have only one abnormal test from the previous list while the other tests are normal; this person would still be diagnosed as having diabetes.

WHAT DOES IT ALL MEAN?

- Diabetes can be diagnosed using multiple tests. Some tests require the person to fast while others do not. This may affect the choice of testing for a specific individual. Any of the tests can be used to diagnose diabetes.
- Abnormal glucose tests should ideally be repeated before the diagnosis of diabetes is made.
- Almost all types of diabetes are diagnosed using the same criteria, with the exception of gestational diabetes, which has special considerations (see "Gestational Diabetes" on page 207).

Risk Factors for Type 1 Diabetes

Risk factors make a person more likely to develop a disease such as diabetes. They can also increase the chance that an existing disease, such as diabetes, will get worse. Where you live, your ethnicity, your family history, and your age may all play a role in defining your risk for type 1 diabetes. Type 1 diabetes accounts for a small fraction of people with diabetes (about 5%).

▶ WHAT YOU NEED TO KNOW

Your Environment

- People who live in Northern Europe may be at higher risk for type 1 diabetes. Interestingly, the highest rates for developing type 1 diabetes have been found in Finland.
- Exposure to certain viruses (such as coxsackie B) may trigger the immune

system to attack the pancreas and lead to type 1 diabetes, but this is still an area of active research.

Your Family History or Genetics

- If the father has type 1 diabetes, there is a 6% chance that his child will develop it too; the risk is less if the mother has type 1 diabetes (2% to 3%).
- If a sibling (brother or sister) has type 1 diabetes, there's a 5% chance a brother or sister will have it too.
- If one identical twin has type 1 diabetes, the other twin (who shares the same genes) has a 30% to 50% chance of having it.
- If a parent and one of her or his children have type 1 diabetes, there is a 30% chance that another child will develop type 1 diabetes too.
- Many different genes likely contribute to type 1 diabetes. Human leukocyte antigen (HLA) genes that have a role in the immune system account for approximately 40% of the genetic risk for the condition. Other genetic variations, such as those in the insulin gene or the protein tyrosine phosphatase gene, may also contribute, but more research is needed.

Your Age or Ethnicity

- Symptoms often appear in elementary or middle school.
- Diagnoses are on the rise among children, including those from racial and ethnic minority groups, such as Hispanics and blacks.
- Once thought of as a disease presenting only in childhood, type 1 diabetes is now being diagnosed in many adults.
- Non-Hispanic whites have a higher risk; Asians have a relatively lower risk.

WHAT DOES IT ALL MEAN?

Many factors likely affect the risk for type 1 diabetes. A mix of genetics and environmental factors may contribute to a person's risk.

Risk Factors for Type 2 Diabetes

Identifying risk factors for type 2 diabetes and an appropriate treatment can potentially reduce the risk of developing diabetes and its complications in the future. Type 2 diabetes accounts for most people (about 90% to 95%) with diabetes.

There are many risk factors for type 2 diabetes. Some of these factors can be changed (for example, being overweight or obese, eating a poor diet, or lacking exercise) while others cannot (for example, age, racial or ethnic background, family history). If one of your parents, siblings, or children (any first-degree relative) has type 2 diabetes, you have a higher than average risk (40% to 50%) of getting it too.

Are You at Risk for Type 2 Diabetes?

1 Are you 45 years or older (even if you don't have symptoms)?
2 If you are a woman, do you have a history of gestational diabetes (diabetes when you were pregnant)?
3 Have you ever had an abnormally high blood glucose test or been told you have prediabetes (see "Testing for Prediabetes" on page 18)?
4 If you're younger than 45 and overweight or obese, take this quiz:
   - Do you have a parent, sibling, or child with diabetes?
   - Are you inactive during the day, with little or no physical activity?
   - Are you African American, Hispanic, Native American, or Asian American?
   - Do you have high blood pressure?
   - Do you have high cholesterol?
   - Are you a woman with polycystic ovarian syndrome (see "Polycystic Ovarian Syndrome" on page 214)?
   - Do you have heart disease?

If you answered yes to one or more of these questions, you could be at risk for diabetes. Contact your health care provider to ask about the need for further testing.

What Common Lifestyle Changes Are Recommended?

- **Body weight** If you are overweight or obese, with a body mass index (BMI) of 25 kilograms per square meter (kg/m^2) or greater (in Asians, 23 kg/m^2 or greater), your chances of developing diabetes are higher. Calculate your BMI using table 6.1. Losing weight by 5% to 7% can dramatically lower your risk.
- **Exercise** Regular exercise—at least 150 minutes a week of moderate-intensity physical activity—can lower your chance of developing diabetes.
- **Healthy diet** You can lower your chance of developing diabetes by limiting processed, calorie-dense food and sugar-sweetened beverages and

monitoring fats. Choose healthy alternatives. The key to a healthy diet is reducing the number of calories you eat, which will help you lose weight.

WHAT DOES IT ALL MEAN?

- There are multiple risk factors for developing type 2 diabetes. Persons with prediabetes are likely to develop type 2 diabetes unless appropriate lifestyle changes similar to those in the Diabetes Prevention Program (see "Testing for Prediabetes" on page 18) are made. Obesity and family history are also common risk factors. Gestational diabetes (see "Gestational Diabetes" on page 207) is a major risk factor for developing type 2 diabetes in women.
- All persons who are 45 years and older should be tested for diabetes. Those who are younger and are obese or overweight with additional risk factors for diabetes should consider being tested.
- Identifying risk factors is important to diagnose prediabetes or diabetes in a timely manner and prevent its complications.

Differences between Type 1 and Type 2 Diabetes

Diagnosing a person's type of diabetes is important because it determines what treatments will work best. There are important differences between type 1 diabetes (fewer than 5% of persons) and type 2 diabetes (90% to 95% of persons). Gestational diabetes is diagnosed for the first time during pregnancy (see "Gestational Diabetes" on page 207). Other types, such as steroid-induced diabetes or unusual genetic forms of diabetes, also exist.

▶ WHAT YOU NEED TO KNOW

Table 2.1. What you need to know about type 1 and type 2 diabetes

	TYPE 1 DIABETES	TYPE 2 DIABETES
Formerly known as . . .	"Juvenile onset" or "insulin-dependent" diabetes.	"Adult onset" or "non-insulin-dependent" diabetes.
Who is diagnosed?	Children and teens, usually with healthy body weight, but also diagnosed in adults.	Usually diagnosed in adults who are overweight or obese but also diagnosed in children.

Table 2.1. (*continued*)

	TYPE 1 DIABETES	TYPE 2 DIABETES
Do other family members have diabetes too?	These people may be the only ones in their family with the disease.	These people often have first-degree relatives with diabetes (parents, siblings, or children).
What causes it?	The person's immune system mistakenly attacks and destroys the insulin-producing (beta) cells of the pancreas. The pancreas can no longer produce any insulin, a hormone needed for controlling blood glucose.	These people can generally still produce insulin, but the body becomes "resistant" to its effects, and insulin is not able to work as well. As a result, blood glucose levels rise. The pancreas tries to produce more insulin to compensate in the early stages, but over time the pancreas "burns out" and eventually stops producing any insulin at all.
What are the risk factors?	Unclear; there may be some environmental risk factors, but a few genetic risk factors have also been identified.	Multiple risk factors include being overweight or obese; belonging to an ethnic minority; history of prediabetes, high blood pressure, high cholesterol, or heart disease; history of gestational diabetes or polycystic ovarian syndrome in women; family history; physical inactivity.
What are the symptoms?	Symptoms include blurry vision, hunger, fatigue, thirstiness, and frequent urination. Unexplained weight loss, nausea, and vomiting are also common symptoms.	Symptoms include blurry vision, hunger, fatigue, thirstiness, and urinating more. Some weight loss may also occur before diagnosis. Symptoms of nerve damage, such as numbness, tingling, or pain in the hands or feet, may already be present at diagnosis.

How is it detected?	Autoantibody tests (such as GAD antibody) and C-peptide measurement (a protein that splits apart from insulin) may clarify whether a person has type 1 diabetes.	There is usually no specific blood test that distinguishes type 2 diabetes. The diagnosis is based on being overweight or obese (but not always) and other risk factors (such as a family history).
How is it treated?	People with type 1 diabetes need to take insulin injections. In the first few months after diagnosis, called the "honeymoon phase," insulin injections might not be needed. But insulin therapy is always needed in the long term.	Some people with type 2 diabetes can manage their blood glucose by reducing their weight and changing their diet. Most others are treated with pills, injectable medicines, or eventually with insulin injections.
What medical emergencies will need hospitalization?	Diabetic ketoacidosis (DKA) is a potentially life-threatening emergency that often occurs at diagnosis due to lack of insulin in the body and buildup of acid in the blood, resulting in tremendous dehydration.	Hyperosmolar hyperglycemia syndrome (HHS) is potentially life-threatening and occurs from having extremely high blood glucose levels, often over 600 mg/dl* (33.3 mmol/L), and is accompanied by tremendous dehydration.
What is the risk of low blood glucose (hypoglycemia)?	In general, the risk of hypoglycemia is high since people with type 1 diabetes are always treated with insulin. Also, since people with type 1 diabetes may not have enough glucagon (a hormone produced by the pancreas that raises blood glucose when needed), low blood glucose levels can occur more frequently and severely.	Generally, the risk of hypoglycemia depends on the type of treatment. It's more likely in persons with type 2 diabetes on pills that stimulate insulin production (that is, sulfonylureas) or on insulin injections. Missed meals and more exercise than usual can also increase the likelihood of hypoglycemia.

*mg/dL = milligrams per deciliter, used to indicate the level of glucose in the blood.

- There are important differences between type 1 diabetes and type 2 diabetes when it comes to risk factors, causes, and whether other family members are affected.
- Diagnosing the type of diabetes is important for appropriate treatment. In general, the symptoms are similar for type 1 and type 2 diabetes.
- Potentially life-threatening *hyperglycemic* (high blood glucose) and *hypoglycemic* (low blood glucose) emergencies can occur in either type of diabetes.

Testing for Prediabetes

Prediabetes occurs when blood glucose levels are higher than normal but not yet high enough to be considered diabetes. Often persons with prediabetes do not have any symptoms, and most people with prediabetes don't know they have it. Prediabetes can lead to heart disease, stroke, nerve damage, and type 2 diabetes, the most common form of diabetes. People with prediabetes may be able to delay or prevent the development of type 2 diabetes with appropriate changes to diet and lifestyle or, in some people, by taking metformin.

▶ WHAT YOU NEED TO KNOW

According to the American Diabetes Association, persons are diagnosed with prediabetes if *any* of the following tests are abnormal:

- **Fasting blood glucose** People who have a mildly high blood glucose after not eating for at least 8 hours have *impaired fasting glucose*. After fasting, the blood glucose levels in a person without diabetes are usually less than 100 mg/dL (5.6 mmol/L). A person with diabetes has blood glucose levels of 126 mg/dL (7.0 mmol/L) or higher. People who don't fit into either category—with levels between 100 and 125 mg/dL (between 5.6 and 6.9 mmol/L)—are described as having prediabetes.
- **OGTT** People who experience an abnormal rise in blood glucose after consuming a concentrated sugar drink have *impaired glucose tolerance*. Health care providers diagnose this condition by testing a person's blood glucose 2 hours after he or she consumes a sweet drink containing 75 grams of glucose. People without diabetes have blood glucose levels less than 140 mg/dL (7.8 mmol/L). A person with diabetes has blood glucose levels 200 mg/dL (11.1 mmol/L) or higher. Persons whose blood glucose levels fall in the

middle, between 140 and 199 mg/dL (between 7.8 and 11.0 mmol/L), have prediabetes.

- **Hemoglobin A1C** People with hemoglobin A1C levels between 5.7% to 6.4% (between 39 to 47 mmol/mol) fall into the "category of high risk for diabetes." People with normal blood glucose levels have hemoglobin A1C levels below 5.7% (39 mmol/mol). People with diabetes have levels 6.5% (48 mmol/mol) or greater. Someone whose A1C levels fall between the two cutoffs are in a category of high risk.

Should I Be Screened for Prediabetes?
Talk to your health care provider, particularly if you
- are 45 years or older;
- are overweight or obese (with a BMI of 25 kg/m^2 or greater; in Asians, 23 kg/m^2 or greater) at any age;
- have a family history of diabetes in a first-degree relative (parents, siblings, children);
- are inactive during the day, with little or no physical activity;
- have a history of gestational diabetes; or
- belong to a minority racial or ethnic group, including Hispanics and African Americans.

Simple online tests are available for you to take and determine if you are at risk for prediabetes or diabetes. For example, the Centers for Disease Control and Prevention (https://www.cdc.gov/diabetes/prevention/pdf/prediabetes test.pdf) and the American Diabetes Association (www.diabetes.org/are-you-at-risk/diabetes-risk-test) each have their own version. Talk to your health care provider if your score indicates that you might be at risk. A blood test will be required to provide a definite diagnosis of prediabetes.

Why Is It Important to Diagnose Prediabetes?
Don't let the "pre" in prediabetes lead you to believe that it's not really a problem. There are steps that you can take now to prevent prediabetes from becoming type 2 diabetes and to reduce the risk of heart attack and stroke. A prediabetes diagnosis does not mean you will definitely develop type 2 diabetes—healthy lifestyle changes or taking metformin can dramatically reduce your risk of developing diabetes and delay its onset. A landmark study called the Diabetes Prevention Program (see "Landmark Studies in Diabetes Care" on page 7) demonstrated that among persons with prediabetes, intensive lifestyle

changes dramatically reduced the development of diabetes by 58% (or approximately half). These changes may include

- eating a healthy diet,
- exercising regularly (for example, 30 minutes of brisk walking per day, 5 days a week), and
- losing weight (7% of body weight, which, for example, would be about 14 pounds in a 200-pound person).

In some cases of prediabetes where lifestyle changes are not feasible or practical, the medication metformin may be prescribed. It is particularly effective for people with severe obesity or a history of gestational diabetes. However, metformin is not currently approved by the Food and Drug Administration for the treatment of prediabetes.

WHAT DOES IT ALL MEAN?

- Many different tests can be used to diagnose prediabetes. These are the same as those used to diagnose diabetes but use lower glucose cutoffs to define an abnormal test.
- Prediabetes is not just a "precursor" state to diabetes. It is a medical condition that is important to diagnose and can be related to the development of multiple medical conditions, such as heart disease, stroke, and even nerve damage.
- Lifestyle changes, including dietary modifications and regular physical activity that result in modest weight loss (7%), can dramatically reduce the development of diabetes in persons with prediabetes. Ask your health care provider about programs based on the Diabetes Prevention Program that may be in your area. Some of these may be covered by insurance.
- Without appropriate lifestyle changes or metformin treatment, many people with prediabetes will develop type 2 diabetes within 5 years. Even more concerning, the majority of people with prediabetes will go on to develop diabetes in their lifetimes.

Latent Autoimmune Diabetes in Adults

In most cases, type 1 diabetes appears in childhood or the early teen years. However, it can also develop in adults and may present up until the eighth or ninth decade of life. This less-common form of diabetes is known as *latent autoimmune diabetes in adults* (LADA). Some expert groups alternatively include this condition under the standard definition of type 1 diabetes as "adult-onset type 1 diabetes."

Is LADA the Same as Type 1 Diabetes Diagnosed in Childhood?

LADA and type 1 diabetes in childhood both occur when the body's immune system attacks the insulin-producing cells of the pancreas. But these conditions differ in several important ways:

- LADA usually develops during adulthood as a slower-onset type 1 diabetes.
- LADA develops more gradually, often without the abrupt and severe rise in blood glucose that occurs when children are first diagnosed with type 1 diabetes.
- Most people with LADA are capable of producing their own insulin when first diagnosed, but many stop producing insulin within a few years of diagnosis. Some may not require insulin or still make enough insulin to more easily control their blood glucose many years later.

Is LADA the Same as Type 2 Diabetes?

No. Though LADA develops during adulthood, it is not the same as type 2 diabetes. The majority of people with LADA are initially misdiagnosed as having type 2 diabetes yet have the presence of autoantibodies. (See "Testing for Autoantibodies" on page 193.) There are important differences between LADA and type 2 diabetes:

- People with LADA are more likely to be of average body weight or underweight, while most people with type 2 diabetes are overweight. However, being overweight does not exclude the possibility of LADA.
- A family history of diabetes is more often absent in people with LADA compared to type 2 diabetes.
- High blood pressure and high cholesterol may or may not be problems for people with LADA.

How Is LADA Treated?

Although LADA may initially appear to respond to treatments for type 2 diabetes, such as lifestyle changes, oral medications, or non-insulin injections, insulin is the recommended treatment. If you are diagnosed with LADA, your provider may recommend daily insulin injections—even if your body can still produce some insulin on its own—to get glucose levels within a healthy range and prevent complications. Some studies suggest that keeping blood glucose levels well managed may also prolong the body's remaining ability to produce at least some insulin.

It's important to follow your health care provider's instructions closely because people with LADA face the risk of having many of the same acute complications as children with type 1 diabetes. They also may experience the long-term complications that affect other people with diabetes, including diseases of the heart, kidneys, nerves, and eyes.

WHAT DOES IT ALL MEAN?

- LADA, or adult-onset type 1 diabetes, is similar to type 1 diabetes diagnosed during childhood in which the body's immune system attacks the pancreas. However, in contrast, LADA results in a slow loss of the ability to produce insulin in adults.
- People with LADA ultimately require treatment with insulin.

Maturity-Onset Diabetes of the Young

Maturity-onset diabetes of the young (MODY) is a distinct type of diabetes. It is different from type 1 and type 2 diabetes. Unlike other types of diabetes, MODY is not caused by damage to the pancreas or an inability of the body to respond to insulin. Rather, MODY occurs when the cells responsible for making insulin in the pancreatic islets—or beta cells—have a genetic defect that causes them not to work as well as they should.

▶ WHAT YOU NEED TO KNOW

This form of diabetes is rare (about 1% to 2% of all people with diabetes) and is almost always caused by a defective gene passed down from parents to their children. In fact, if one parent has the disease, there's a 50/50 chance the child will develop it too. Most people with MODY are often first mistakenly diagnosed with type 1 diabetes and treated with insulin but, if correctly diagnosed, can be treated with oral medications or diet, similar to type 2 diabetes.

At What Age Does MODY Typically Develop?

People with MODY begin to develop mild and often asymptomatic diabetes during childhood, the teen years, or in their early 20s—but almost always before age 25. Most children have a normal body weight, and people with MODY do not initially require insulin treatment.

How Is It Diagnosed?

If you have diabetes and your provider suspects MODY, he or she will look closely at your family medical history to see if at least three generations—usually your parents, grandparents, or great-grandparents—developed high blood glucose levels before age 25.

There are different subtypes of MODY, each one caused by a mutation in a specific gene. Identifying the genetic defect is important to guide treatment, and the risk of long-term complications may differ. For instance, those with the glucokinase defect do not generally require treatment for diabetes or develop complications since fasting blood glucose levels are only slightly higher than usual.

What Treatments Are Available?

Your health care provider will work with you to create an individualized treatment plan. Depending on which subtype of MODY you have inherited, the provider might initially recommend anything from a balanced diet and exercise to an oral pill. Fortunately, several treatments are available to help keep blood glucose levels within a healthy range.

▶ WHAT YOU NEED TO KNOW

- MODY is a distinct type of diabetes caused by a defective gene. The disease is passed on from generation to generation and usually becomes apparent before age 25. There is a 50% chance of a parent passing on MODY to his or her child.
- Depending on the type of gene defect, oral pills may be needed to keep glucose levels in the normal range. It is important to identify the genetic defect since certain medications (for example, sulfonylureas) might be preferred. Insulin is not necessarily needed.
- Genetic testing may be offered for family members.

Cystic Fibrosis–Related Diabetes

Cystic fibrosis is an inherited disease caused by a genetic mutation in the *CFTR* gene. The mutation blocks the normal flow of salt and water and can affect multiple organs in the body, most commonly the lungs. This disease can also cause problems with the pancreas, the organ that makes insulin, making it difficult to control blood glucose.

When diabetes develops in a person with cystic fibrosis, it's considered neither type 1 nor type 2 diabetes. Rather, it's given its own name: *cystic fibrosis–related diabetes* (CFRD). CFRD is the most common disease-related condition occurring in people with cystic fibrosis.

The genetic defect that causes cystic fibrosis has multiple effects, both in the pancreas as a whole and in the *pancreatic islets* (that make insulin and other hormones). The thick mucus that is characteristic of cystic fibrosis may lead to scarring of the pancreas and reduce the ability to digest certain foods and vitamins. The insulin-producing cells in the pancreatic islets may also be affected and stop making enough insulin (causing high blood glucose levels). When people with cystic fibrosis develop diabetes, their bodies can usually still respond to insulin normally. People with CFRD can get many of the usual complications of diabetes, such as eye disease and kidney disease, but perhaps the most common complication of CFRD is a worsening of the lung disease in cystic fibrosis. Therefore, treating the diabetes is particularly important to preserve lung function.

At What Age Does Diabetes Develop in People with Cystic Fibrosis?

People with cystic fibrosis are more likely to develop diabetes as they get older. About 20% of adolescents and 40% to 50% of adults with cystic fibrosis will have CFRD.

How Is Cystic Fibrosis–Related Diabetes Diagnosed?

Many experts recommend testing everyone with cystic fibrosis annually for diabetes beginning at the age of 10 years. In addition, if you have cystic fibrosis and develop any of the symptoms or signs of diabetes (thirstiness, frequent urination, difficulty gaining or maintaining weight, unexpected declines in lung function, slower than expected growth, or delayed puberty), your health care provider will recommend testing for diabetes. Typically, cystic fibrosis–related diabetes is diagnosed with an oral glucose tolerance test (measuring glucose values after ingesting a fixed amount of glucose), as other tests (such as a hemoglobin A1C blood test) are not as accurate in cystic fibrosis.

What Are the Treatment Options?

People with CFRD usually don't respond as well to oral diabetes medications. Rather, diabetes in people with CFRD is best treated with insulin. Often, lower doses are needed compared to type 1 diabetes. Either long-acting insulin (taken once or twice daily) or rapid-acting insulin (taken at meals), or both, may be beneficial. Sometimes insulin is needed only temporarily. The goals of diabetes care are similar to other types of diabetes except for the dietary recommendations (see below). Health care providers might recommend regular exercise and routine checkup appointments with diabetes specialists and educators.

Should People with Cystic Fibrosis Eat a Modified Diet?

No. In fact, that's one of the major differences between people with cystic fibrosis and other people with diabetes. People with cystic fibrosis are often underweight and have congestion in their lungs. The work of breathing burns a lot of energy. As a result, providers don't usually limit the number of carbs that people with cystic fibrosis eat. In fact, people with cystic fibrosis are encouraged to continue their high-calorie, high-protein, high-fat diet so they can gain and maintain a healthy weight. The main modification is that they are asked to avoid pure sugars (such as sodas) and instead eat a combination of complex and simple carbohydrates mixed with protein and fat. This is different than other forms of diabetes, in which people are usually asked to monitor their carbohydrates. Insulin treatment often needs to be adjusted with any changes in diet.

WHAT DOES IT ALL MEAN?

- Adolescents and adults with cystic fibrosis should be monitored carefully for signs of diabetes and should have routine diabetes screening tests.
- If a person with cystic fibrosis has trouble maintaining or gaining weight, is not growing as quickly as expected, or has difficulty breathing for no apparent reason, be sure to ask the provider about getting screened for diabetes.

Diabetes after Pancreatic Surgery

One of the main roles of the islets (the groups of hormone-producing cells) in the pancreas is to make insulin, which is necessary for processing glucose in the body. If a person has surgery to remove part of the pancreas, this can lead to diabetes. Knowing the type of surgery and the person's other diabetes risk factors can help determine his or her chances of developing diabetes following pancreas surgery.

▶ WHAT YOU NEED TO KNOW

Removing all or part of the pancreas is a treatment for pancreatic cancer, pancreatitis with chronic pain, and a host of other conditions.

The pancreas produces the hormone insulin, which lowers blood glucose levels. Regardless of whether someone had diabetes before surgery, removing all or part of the pancreas can lead to diabetes, also called *postpancreatectomy diabetes*.

How Can I Prepare for This Surgery?

It is important to discuss the expected outcomes, including the possibility

Table 2.2. Common pancreatic surgeries and the risk of developing diabetes

NAME OF SURGERY	HOW IT WORKS	POSSIBILITY OF DIABETES
Total pancreatectomy	The entire pancreas is removed.	Certain. Without the pancreas, the body is unable to make its own insulin, so the patient will need multiple daily injections of insulin.
Partial pancreatectomy or near-total pancreatectomy	Only part of the pancreas is removed.	When nearly all (about 95%) of the pancreas is removed, almost all people will require multiple daily insulin injections. If a smaller part of the pancreas is removed, the likelihood of needing insulin injections is less.
Pancreaticoduodenectomy ("Whipple")	A small part of the pancreas known as the "head" is removed. This is a very common type of pancreatic surgery.	Up to half of people who didn't have diabetes before the surgery will develop diabetes after the procedure.
Distal pancreatectomy	A small part of the pancreas known as the "tail" is removed.	Up to one-third of people who didn't have diabetes before the surgery will develop diabetes after the procedure.

of worsening diabetes or developing new-onset diabetes, before scheduling pancreas surgery. Time should be taken to understand how daily activities will likely change. In the days or weeks before surgery, people scheduled to have their entire pancreas removed (total pancreatectomy) or who are at risk for developing diabetes after pancreas surgery should practice using a home blood glucose meter, counting the carbohydrates in each meal, and reviewing how to calculate doses of insulin.

Does Pancreatic Surgery Always Lead to Diabetes?
It can be difficult to know in advance if a person will develop diabetes, as this

depends on many factors, including how much and what part of the pancreas is removed. Some people will require insulin injections, and some might not develop diabetes at all.

On the other hand, people who have their entire pancreas removed will no longer make their own insulin. They will definitely develop diabetes and will need multiple daily insulin injections, beginning immediately after the procedure (table 2.2).

How Soon after Surgery Will I Know If I Have Diabetes?

People who have their entire pancreas removed will always develop diabetes and will require multiple daily insulin injections immediately after surgery. People who have only a part of their pancreas removed will receive instructions on how to measure their blood glucose levels in the days after surgery to determine if they will need insulin.

Because most people don't eat or drink much during the recovery period, the amount of insulin needed will change daily until the patient regains a full appetite. After discharge, people with postpancreatectomy diabetes should stay in close contact with their providers to make sure their doses of insulin are enough to keep their blood glucose within healthy levels.

If I Develop Diabetes after Pancreatic Surgery, How Will It Be Treated?

Every person who has pancreatic surgery and develops diabetes should schedule a follow-up visit with a diabetes specialist, known as an *endocrinologist*, and a diabetes educator or dietitian, as appropriate. An individual treatment plan will be developed based on each person's overall health and glucose levels.

WHAT DOES IT ALL MEAN?

- Removing the entire pancreas will result in diabetes that must be treated with multiple daily insulin injections immediately after surgery. Pancreatic enzyme replacement is also required to aid with digestion.
- The removal of a portion of the pancreas may lead to diabetes. People who have other risk factors for diabetes before surgery (for example, prediabetes) are more likely to develop diabetes after a partial pancreatectomy.
- After surgery, a diabetes specialist can work with people who develop postpancreatectomy diabetes to set goals for blood glucose management and to educate family members and caregivers.

- People with diabetes before surgery will likely need increased medication doses after surgery and will often require insulin.

Steroid-Induced Diabetes

Steroid-induced diabetes refers to prolonged high blood glucose levels due to glucocorticoid therapies (steroids) prescribed for another medical condition (such as asthma or chronic obstructive pulmonary disease). It is often, but not always, a temporary condition that resolves after the steroid therapy is stopped.

▶ WHAT YOU NEED TO KNOW

Many hospitalized patients and people receiving organ transplants are treated with steroid drugs, such as hydrocortisone or prednisone. These drugs are used to reduce inflammation and suppress the immune system, but they can also result in high blood glucose levels or, eventually, steroid-induced diabetes in those at high risk. The symptoms share similarities with those of other types of diabetes and include

- urinating frequently;
- feeling hungrier than usual;
- excessive thirst;
- feeling tired, even after a full night's sleep; and
- infections that don't seem to heal.

Who Is at Risk?

Up to half of all hospitalized patients who take high doses of steroids and have other risk factors for diabetes will develop high blood glucose levels. Persons who already have diabetes often find it difficult to control their blood glucose when they take steroids. Persons in the intensive care unit are at higher risk and are more likely to develop high blood glucose levels when taking steroids compared with other hospitalized patients.

If This Condition Is Temporary, Why Should I Notify My Health Care Provider?

People with normal blood glucose levels often have a shorter hospital stay, develop fewer infections, and recover more quickly than people with severely high blood glucose levels who require treatment to lower them. A history of steroid-induced diabetes usually indicates the presence of other risk factors for developing diabetes.

What Treatments Are Available?

The treatment for steroid-induced diabetes is insulin therapy (particularly in the hospital) and sometimes pills after discharge.

When Should I Call My Health Care Provider for an Update?

Make sure your health care provider knows as soon as you stop taking steroids or have a change in the steroid dose. It's very important that your provider reduces your diabetes medications when the steroid dose is lowered to prevent dangerous drops in blood glucose. If your blood glucose level doesn't return to normal after you stop taking steroids, notify your provider. Sometimes those with steroid-induced diabetes who were already at high risk continue to have diabetes even after the steroids are stopped and require lifelong treatment.

WHAT DOES IT ALL MEAN?

- Steroids can increase blood glucoses levels, even in people without diabetes, particularly in the hospital setting. Usually, if blood glucose levels rise in a person treated with steroids, it indicates the presence of other risk factors for developing diabetes.
- People who already have diabetes should be more cautious if a health care provider prescribes a steroid medication, such as hydrocortisone or prednisone, or even steroid (or "cortisone") injections for joint pain. If this happens be sure to ask your provider about possibly increasing your diabetes medications to prevent a rise in blood glucose and what to do if glucose levels run high afterward.
- Any dose changes in steroid-containing medications can affect the need for glucose-lowering therapies, and these must be adjusted accordingly in consultation with a medical provider.

Chapter 3

GENERAL ASPECTS OF DIABETES

MONITORING BLOOD GLUCOSE LEVELS
Self-Monitoring of Blood Glucose

Self-monitoring of blood glucose (SMBG) refers to the process of home blood glucose testing by persons with diabetes. It is a tool to help persons with diabetes better understand patterns of high and low blood glucose levels during the day. Information from SMBG testing is also used to adjust diabetes medications.

▶ WHAT YOU NEED TO KNOW

Some Key Facts

1 Blood glucose is monitored at home using a small handheld machine called a *glucose meter* (figure 3.1).

2 Persons with type 1 diabetes usually need to measure their blood glucose level at least four times a day. Persons with type 2 diabetes who take insulin also need to measure their glucose levels regularly, as recommended by their health care provider. The frequency of glucose monitoring for persons with type 2 diabetes not taking insulin is individualized but usually at least once a day, often in the morning upon awakening and sometimes before other meals and bedtime.

3 Most glucose meters require a drop of blood from a pinprick of the person's finger. The blood glucose value is then displayed on the glucose meter's screen.

4 The home blood glucose test is useful because the person with diabetes can perform it anywhere and at any time.

5 The dates, times, and blood glucose readings are all stored in the meter's memory, which can often hold a few months of readings. These results can be downloaded onto a computer and used by people with diabetes and their providers to make dosing adjustments.

6 The test strips that come with the meter can give inaccurate readings if they are stored in locations that are too hot or cold or if they expire. It's important to store the test strips as carefully as you would any medication. Glucose test strips should never be reused, and purchasing preowned test strips can result in false results. Each specific glucose meter has its own recommended test strips; *if others are used, the glucose meter may fail to provide results or give incorrect glucose readings.*

7 The test strips can give inaccurate readings if a person's blood glucose level is very high or very low. Persons with diabetes should check with their health care provider if they receive a reading far outside the normal range.

8 If lotion or food residue is on the skin, blood taken from that area may give an inaccurate reading. First, wash the area or swab it with alcohol to make sure the skin is clean. Hand sanitizers may not always be adequate to clean the skin used for testing.

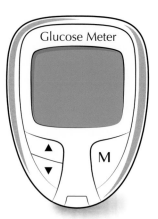

3.1 Glucose meters are small handheld devices used to test your blood glucose at home. A small blood sample is obtained, usually from your fingertip. From this blood sample, a blood glucose level can be determined. © 2018, Johns Hopkins University, Art as Applied to Medicine

WHAT DOES IT ALL MEAN?

- SMBG is a convenient way for people with diabetes to monitor their blood glucose levels at school, work, or on the road. The test results can help the health care provider and person with diabetes better manage glucose levels. The amount of blood needed for the test is minimal and usually causes no significant discomfort when performed appropriately.

- The frequency of SMBG differs for each person and depends on the type of diabetes and use of insulin therapy.
- When used regularly, SMBG can lead to the early identification of potentially dangerous situations, such as diabetic ketoacidosis (see "Diabetic Ketoacidosis" on page 35) or severe hypoglycemia (low blood glucose), and facilitate timely and appropriate treatment.

The Dawn Phenomenon

The *dawn phenomenon* describes a daily rise in blood glucose values that many persons with diabetes experience in the early morning hours. Understanding this phenomenon can help improve blood glucose management.

▶ WHAT YOU NEED TO KNOW

People with diabetes know that it takes constant watchfulness to keep blood glucose levels in check. Yet despite their best efforts, more than half of all people with diabetes experience a sudden surge in blood glucose every morning—even though they didn't eat anything overnight.

Why Does This Happen?

During certain stages of sleep, your body releases hormones to help promote the growth and maintenance of cells in the body. One of these hormones, aptly named *growth hormone*, reduces the sensitivity of your muscles and liver to insulin (meaning insulin doesn't work as well during that time). Other hormones, such as cortisol, tend to peak in the morning and can further raise blood glucose levels. As a result, people with diabetes are more likely than others to experience a sudden surge in blood glucose levels between four and eight o'clock in the morning. This is the dawn phenomenon.

Who Is at Risk?
- The dawn phenomenon is most frequent and noticeable in people with poorly managed blood glucose levels.
- People with type 1 diabetes are at greatest risk in the initial years following their diagnosis.
- People with type 2 diabetes tend to experience the dawn phenomenon more often as their disease progresses.

How Is It Diagnosed and Treated?
- If your blood glucose is routinely high when you awaken in the morning,

your provider might ask you to record your blood glucose levels before bed, overnight (such as at 2:00 or 3:00 a.m.), and when you wake up. The dawn phenomenon should not be confused with the gradual rise in blood glucose that occurs as a dose of intermediate- or long-acting insulin wears off throughout the early hours of the morning.

- People with type 1 diabetes should avoid late-night snacking and might need to adjust their dose of long-acting insulin to prevent the dawn phenomenon. People with an insulin pump might be advised to increase the rate of insulin delivery during the early morning hours for a short period of time.
- People with type 2 diabetes who experience the dawn phenomenon should consider decreasing the amount of carbohydrates in their evening meal—or eating an earlier evening meal—so their blood glucose levels are not too high before bedtime. If dietary changes are not effective, the health care provider might prescribe an intermediate- or long-acting insulin (for example, NPH, glargine, detemir, or degludec) to take before bedtime or physical activity in the evening, such as a walk after dinner.

WHAT DOES IT ALL MEAN?

The early-morning rise in blood glucose levels called the dawn phenomenon is common in people with diabetes. The health care provider may adjust the dose of bedtime insulin or the early-morning insulin pump settings to help combat the dawn phenomenon in people with type 1 or type 2 diabetes treated with insulin. For people with type 2 diabetes, if the rise in early-morning glucose is not managed with dietary changes in the evening, the addition of an intermediate- or long-acting insulin may be recommended.

Hemoglobin A1C Testing

Hemoglobin A1C, also known as *A1C* or *glycosylated hemoglobin*, is a test that indirectly estimates the average blood glucose levels over the past 3 months. Blood glucose levels fluctuate from hour to hour, day to day, but the A1C level reflects the overall average and is the best test to monitor longer-term blood glucose control. Higher A1C levels are related to the development of complications in persons with diabetes.

Hemoglobin (the protein that carries oxygen) in red blood cells gradually be-comes coated with glucose molecules from the blood—and more so in people with diabetes. The hemoglobin A1C test works by measuring the percentage of hemoglobin with glucose molecules attached. In people without diabetes, A1C levels range from about 4% to 5.7% or 20 to 39 millimoles per mole (mmol/mol).

The A1C test is an important tool for diagnosing and monitoring diabetes (see "Diagnosing Diabetes" on page 11). After diagnosis, most people with dia-betes should take the A1C test every 3 months, but the test might be spaced to every 6 months for people with consistently good levels.

Optimal A1C levels to reduce the risk of developing complications in most nonpregnant persons with diabetes are less than 7% (53 mmol/mol), though older persons with multiple medications and limited mobility may have less stringent goals of lower than 7.5% or 8.5% (58 or 69 mmol/mol). Levels higher than 9% usually suggest overall poor blood glucose management. In younger people with a new diagnosis of diabetes who are otherwise healthy, A1C goals may be set at less than 6.5% (48 mmol/mol).

Table 3.1 illustrates how A1C levels relate to average blood glucose, which is measured in mil-limoles per liter (mmol/L) in many countries outside the United States and milligrams per deciliter (mg/dL) within the United States. In general, an A1C level of 7% (53 mmol/mol) reflects an average blood glu-

Table 3.1. A1C level and estimated average blood glucose levels

A1C (%)	BLOOD GLUCOSE (MG/DL)	BLOOD GLUCOSE (MMOL/L)
6	126	7.0
7	154	8.6
8	183	10.2
9	212	11.8
10	240	13.4
11	269	14.9
12	298	16.5

Note: mg/dL = milligrams per deciliter; mmol/L = millimoles per liter.

cose level of 154 mg/dL (8.6 mmol/L). Every increase of 1% (11 mmol/mol) in A1C reflects a higher average blood glucose level by about 30 mg/dL (1.7 mmol/L), while every decrease of 1% (11 mmol/mol) reflects a lower average blood glucose level by about 30 mg/dL (1.7 mmol/L).

The A1C test can be used in most people with diabetes. However, in people who have abnormal red blood cells (such as with sickle cell disease) or use medications that interfere with the assay (such as large doses of aspirin), other tests to measure average blood glucose levels may be needed; for example, fructosamine. A1C levels may be falsely low—that is, underestimate average blood glucose levels—in people with HIV. A1C may also differ by race and ethnicity, but it remains controversial whether this is related to true differences in average blood glucose levels. To reduce variation in the measurement of A1C, laboratories are recommended to use a National Glycohemoglobin Standardization Program (commonly known as NGSP) certified method.

WHAT DOES IT ALL MEAN?

- If there is one number that all persons with diabetes should know, it is their A1C level. The A1C level is directly related to the risk of complications from diabetes (eye disease, nerve damage, kidney disease, and likely heart disease and stroke). Getting the A1C to target can dramatically reduce the risk of developing these issues.
- The A1C is a weighted average of glucose over the past 3 months; glucose levels in the most recent few weeks will have a greater impact on the A1C value.
- The A1C goal for each person with diabetes needs to be individualized in discussion with a health care provider; for most nonpregnant adults, the goal is less than 7% (53 mmol/mol), according to the American Diabetes Association. Some other professional societies recommend a goal A1C of less than 6.5% (48 mmol/mol). However, people who are older or have multiple other chronic medical conditions may have A1C goals that are higher (such as less than 7.5% to 8.5% or 58 to 69 mmol/mol).

HYPERGLYCEMIC (HIGH BLOOD GLUCOSE) EMERGENCIES
Diabetic Ketoacidosis

People with type 1 diabetes can't produce any insulin on their own, and the body is unable to process carbohydrates from food. Without insulin treatment, glucose in the blood rises dangerously high (above 250 mg/dL or 13.9 mmol/L but usually much higher). In less than 24 hours, the blood can accumulate the breakdown products of fat (which are used as an alternative source of energy) called *ketones*. These ketones appear in the patient's blood and urine, signaling the onset of a potentially life-threatening condition called *diabetic ketoacidosis*, or DKA.

▶ WHAT YOU NEED TO KNOW

Who Is at Risk for DKA?

- Children, teenagers, and adults who do not yet realize they have type 1 diabetes are at high risk for DKA. As you might imagine, DKA is commonly the first presenting symptom for people who have type 1 diabetes but haven't been diagnosed. These people are not yet taking insulin and may not notice the warning signs of high blood glucose.
- People who normally take insulin for type 1 diabetes but
  - skip injections of insulin or miscalculate and underdose insulin repeatedly;
  - stop taking insulin for any reason because of loss of motivation, depression, simply forgetting, or not being able to afford their medications;
  - are using an insulin pump that malfunctions and is not fixed in a timely manner;
  - develop an underlying illness ranging from something as mild as a urinary tract infection to a major event, such as a heart attack. Persons with type 1 diabetes should alert their health care provider if they have a severe or nonhealing infection to get appropriate treatment and reduce the risk of DKA.
- In rare cases, DKA can affect people with type 2 diabetes. This may occur in people diagnosed with diabetes for the first time or who have had the disease for many years, are taking insulin because their body no longer produces enough of the hormone on its own, or who have a severe underlying illness. Persons from high-risk minority groups (that is, African Americans or Hispanics) with type 2 diabetes are more likely to have DKA.

What Are the Signs and Symptoms of DKA?

If you notice these signs or symptoms, seek medical attention:

- Dry mouth
- Slow or very fast heart rate
- Rapid breathing
- Fruity-smelling breath

- Extreme thirst
- Urinating more than usual
- Feeling dehydrated even though you are drinking often
- Feeling tired or lethargic
- Abdominal pain, nausea, and vomiting
- Coma

How Is DKA Treated?

People with DKA are usually admitted to the hospital's intensive care unit (ICU) for close watching as they are treated and recover. These people are extremely dehydrated and must receive intravenous (IV) fluids. The health care provider will give IV insulin to lower blood glucose and reduce the amount of acid in the blood. Blood tests every 1 to 4 hours will monitor the person's blood glucose and electrolytes to make sure they return to normal. Once the person's blood glucose levels improve and the blood no longer has excess acid, the person will be transitioned to insulin injections that can be taken at home, and the IV insulin will be stopped.

WHAT DOES IT ALL MEAN?

Diabetic ketoacidosis is a medical emergency. Sometimes this is a person's first sign of type 1 diabetes; other times this happens if a person stops taking insulin or doesn't take enough. Without proper treatment DKA can lead to coma, swelling of the brain, and even death. If you notice symptoms of DKA, call your health care provider immediately and go to the nearest emergency room. After recovery, work with the health care team to create a plan for preventing another emergency.

Hyperosmolar Hyperglycemic State

People with severely uncontrolled type 2 diabetes can have a dangerous rise in blood glucose levels known as *hyperosmolar hyperglycemic state* (HHS), usually over several days to weeks.

▶ WHAT YOU NEED TO KNOW

Who Is at Risk for HHS?

This condition—and the enormous dehydration that accompanies it—occurs most often in older persons with type 2 diabetes, including nursing home residents. However, any person with very high blood glucose levels is at high risk for developing HHS. People are likely to develop HHS if they forget to take their medicines or develop an underlying illness. This illness can range from something as mild as a urinary tract infection to a major event, such as a heart attack. People with type 2 diabetes should alert their health care provider as soon as they become ill because of the risk of HHS.

What Are the Symptoms of HHS?

People with HHS have extremely high blood glucose levels, often over 600 mg/dL (33.3 mmol/L). If you notice any of these signs or symptoms, seek medical attention:

- Dry mouth
- Cool hands and feet
- Fast heart rate
- Low blood pressure
- Sensation of thirst
- Frequent urination
- Nausea, vomiting, or stomachache
- Mental changes, including confusion, slurred speech, or weakness on one side of the body (similar to the symptoms of a stroke)
- Coma

How Is HHS Treated?

People with HHS are usually admitted to the hospital's ICU because they must be watched very closely as they receive therapy and recover. These people are extremely dehydrated and must be treated with large amounts of IV fluids to help bring blood glucose down to healthy levels. As the person with diabetes is rehydrated, the health care provider will give IV insulin to lower blood glucose levels. Blood tests every 1 to 4 hours will continue to monitor blood glucose and electrolytes to ensure they return to normal. Once the person's blood glucose levels improve and they are properly rehydrated, he or she will be transitioned back to a regular diabetes treatment regimen to be taken at home.

WHAT DOES IT ALL MEAN?

Hyperosmolar hyperglycemic state is a medical emergency for people with type 2 diabetes. Though the condition gradually develops over the course of days or weeks, prompt treatment is extremely important. Unfortunately, one of every five people with HHS does not survive without timely treatment. If you notice signs or symptoms of HHS, call your health care provider immediately and go to the nearest emergency room. After recovery, work together with your health care providers to prevent another emergency. It is important to monitor blood glucose regularly at home, to take medications as directed, and to eat and drink on a regular basis.

HYPOGLYCEMIA (LOW BLOOD GLUCOSE)
Prevention and Treatment of Hypoglycemia

Most people with diabetes, at some time, experience the symptoms that occur when blood glucose levels fall below normal—a condition known as *hypoglycemia*. For many people with diabetes, the symptoms of hypoglycemia start to occur at a level of 70 mg/dL (3.9 mmol/L) or less, but this level may differ for each person.

▶ WHAT YOU NEED TO KNOW

Though hypoglycemia can be common and occur repeatedly in some people with diabetes, symptoms of low blood glucose should always be taken seriously. You may have one or more of the early symptoms listed here (figure 3.2):

Early signs of hypoglycemia: sweating, shakiness, racing heartbeat, flushed face, anxiety, irritability, or hunger pangs.

Late signs of hypoglycemia: headaches, blurred vision, sleepiness, dizziness, lightheadedness, confusion, difficulty speaking or eating, seizures, or coma.

However, sometimes persons with repeated bouts of low blood glucose eventually don't feel any symptoms, a problem called *hypoglycemia unawareness*. A continuous glucose monitor may be helpful for these persons. A critically low blood glucose level is considered to be less than 54 mg/dL (3.0 mmol/L) and can lead to severe neurological symptoms, such as confusion or coma.

What Causes Low Blood Glucose?

In most cases, low blood glucose results from overtreatment, such as taking too much diabetes medication. Insulin and sulfonylureas (and meglitinides) are the medications most commonly associated with hypoglycemia. Delaying or skipping a meal can also deprive the body of glucose and lead to hypoglycemia. Eat balanced meals throughout the day and always keep a snack on hand, particularly if you are on these medications.

Physical activity doesn't just burn calories, it also burns blood glucose. Hypoglycemia can occur if physical activity is increased but the diet or medication

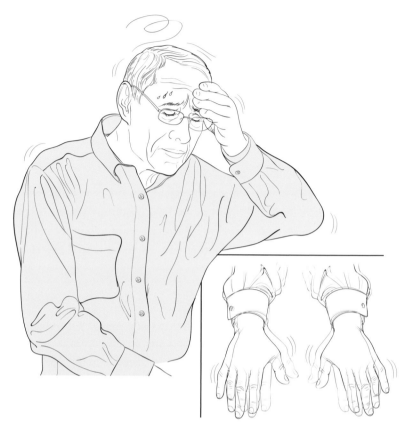

3.2 Feeling sweaty, shaky, hungry, weak, or anxious are all possible early signs of hypoglycemia. Treating a low blood glucose level at the first sign of symptoms is important to prevent the more severe late effects of hypoglycemia. © 2018, Johns Hopkins University, Art as Applied to Medicine

is not appropriately adjusted (such as taking snacks or decreasing medication doses).

Drinking alcohol (without food) or having an illness are other situations in which hypoglycemia is more likely to occur, and precautions to prevent low blood glucose levels should be taken (see "Special Considerations during Sick Days" on page 49).

How Can I Prevent Low Blood Glucose?

- If you often experience low blood glucose, ask your health care provider if setting a higher goal for your A1C level may be appropriate.
- If you've had low blood glucose levels, consider wearing a medical alert

bracelet so that others will know that you have diabetes in the event of an emergency.

- Keep a fast-acting carbohydrate in your bag, office desk drawer, car, bedside table, and other places for easy access. Good options include hard candy, fruit juice, or glucose paste or tablets. Snacks with about 15 grams of carbohydrates are good to correct hypoglycemia.
- Monitor your blood glucose regularly so that low levels can be corrected before symptoms progress.
- These precautions are also important to prevent low blood glucose levels while driving.
- Own an emergency home glucagon kit, particularly if you are on insulin and have a history of hypoglycemia. Glucagon injection is an emergency medicine used to treat severe hypoglycemia in persons with diabetes who have passed out or cannot take anything by mouth.
- For specific details on how to treat hypoglycemia at home, see "Overnight Hypoglycemia" on page 43.

WHAT DOES IT ALL MEAN?

Hypoglycemia usually occurs at some point in persons with diabetes and is commonly related to overtreatment (especially when taking too much insulin or other pills that stimulate insulin production, such as sulfonylureas), delaying or skipping meals, or exercising more than usual. Checking blood glucose levels as recommended can help prevent episodes of hypoglycemia before they happen. If symptoms of hypoglycemia occur, take a fast-acting snack that has 15 grams of carbohydrates to boost your glucose level, and let your health care provider know.

Hypoglycemia after Meals

Low blood glucose doesn't just affect people with diabetes. Almost anyone can have glucose levels drop. But recurring bouts of low blood glucose levels after meals (below 70 mg/dL or 3.9 mmol/L) could signal a condition called *reactive* or *prandial* hypoglycemia.

▶ WHAT YOU NEED TO KNOW

Because even healthy people can have low blood glucose levels after meals on occasion, some experts question whether reactive hypoglycemia is a true medical concern or simply a normal part of life. Either way, low blood glucose is easy to treat: in most cases, a small carbohydrate-containing snack will boost your blood glucose to a normal level.

Why Does It Happen?

Your blood glucose level might drop after a meal for several reasons. Not all of them signal a serious health problem:

- Reactive hypoglycemia can occur in people who are becoming resistant to insulin but do not yet have type 2 diabetes. In these people, the pancreas might overestimate the amount of insulin needed and inadvertently release too much in response to carbohydrate-containing meals.
- After weight-loss surgery, for example, the body requires less insulin than it used to—but sometimes the pancreas doesn't adjust to this change right away. It may be used to secreting large amounts of insulin after meals. Following surgery, the pancreas might release too much insulin after eating carbohydrates, causing a person's blood glucose to drop.
- In most cases, reactive hypoglycemia is not a cause of concern and can be treated with simple dietary modifications.

How Will I Know If I Have Reactive Hypoglycemia?

People who regularly have symptoms of low blood glucose—including hunger, trembling fingers, heart palpitations, weakness, anxiety, or sweating—a few hours after they eat should describe these symptoms to their health care provider. Because many of these symptoms can be caused by other conditions, it's important to confirm that they are due to low blood glucose levels.

Your health care provider may suggest a *mixed meal test*, where you'll eat a meal containing mostly carbs and fat with a small amount of protein or an oral glucose tolerance test (where you'll consume a carbohydrate-containing sugary drink). The provider will then measure your blood glucose at regular intervals for a few hours. If your blood glucoses are indeed low, the provider will give you a small carb-containing snack and monitor your blood glucose to see if it returns to normal.

How Is This Condition Treated?

If you are diagnosed with reactive hypoglycemia, you might consider keeping a log of your blood glucose levels throughout the day so that you can predict when a drop is about to occur. The following tips might also prove helpful:

- Meet with a dietitian to create a healthy meal plan.

- Eat more frequent, small meals while moderating carbohydrate content.
- Add more protein and fiber to your diet.
- Avoid simple sugars, such as regular soda, fruit juices, candy, or concentrated sweets.
- Eat a small carb-containing snack about 30 minutes before your blood glucose is expected to drop.
- If changes to your diet aren't effective, ask your provider about medicines to prevent low blood glucose. In some cases, providers prescribe medicines such as acarbose to delay the digestion of starches and glucoses from foods.

WHAT DOES IT ALL MEAN?

A drop in blood glucose after a meal—termed *reactive hypoglycemia*—is generally not caused by a worrisome condition. Modifying your diet can help prevent these episodes. While reactive hypoglycemia is sometimes an early sign of type 2 diabetes, in other cases the symptoms usually do not worsen or will resolve.

Overnight Hypoglycemia

When blood glucose levels fall low (that is, below 70 mg/dL or 3.9 mmol/L) while a person is sleeping at night, she or he experiences a condition called *nocturnal hypoglycemia*. The symptoms of low blood glucose levels at night are not always the same as during waking hours.

▶ WHAT YOU NEED TO KNOW

Who Is at Risk?

Nocturnal hypoglycemia can affect people who

- are treated with insulin;
- skip meals, particularly dinner;
- exercise before bedtime;
- drink alcohol before bedtime;
- have recently changed their diabetes medications or increased their doses; or
- have previously experienced nocturnal hypoglycemia.

What Are the Warning Signs?

- Restless, irritable sleep

- Hot, clammy, or sweaty skin
- Trembling or shaking
- Changes in breathing (suddenly breathing fast or slow)
- Racing heartbeat
- Sleep disturbances such as nightmares or crying out at night
- Damp sheets or pajamas from sweating excessively overnight
- Feeling tired or confused upon awakening
- Waking with a headache

Health care providers are most concerned about patients who sleep through these symptoms without noticing them.

What Should I Do If This Happens?

People with diabetes and their partners or roommates should learn to recognize the signs of nighttime hypoglycemia. Be prepared! Ask your provider for an emergency glucagon kit. This kit contains a fast-acting medication that can be injected by a partner or roommate to increase blood glucose levels if the person with diabetes can't treat himself or herself safely. Do not put anything into a person's mouth if she or he is unconscious or unable to sit up. Follow these steps:

- If a person cannot be awakened: Call 911 immediately. If the patient has a home glucagon kit, the partner or roommate can follow the instructions to fill the syringe and inject the medicine under the patient's skin or in the muscle (such as the arm, abdomen, or leg) before the ambulance arrives.
- If the person is awake and can sit without support: Give 15 grams of a fast-acting carbohydrate source, such as 4 ounces of juice or regular soda. Other good options include hard candy or glucose paste or tablets, which can be purchased at most pharmacies. Recheck the blood glucose 15 minutes later, particularly if symptoms haven't improved, to ensure it isn't falling further. The person should then eat a snack or meal shortly afterward to prevent further lows.

WHAT DOES IT ALL MEAN?

Nocturnal hypoglycemia can be particularly dangerous since the sleeping individual may not always detect the symptoms of low blood glucose. Learning to recognize the symptoms of nocturnal hypoglycemia, by both people with diabetes and anyone who lives with them, is particularly important. For some people, a continuous glucose monitor at night may help to prevent repeated episodes of nocturnal hypoglycemia.

ROUTINE CARE AND VACCINATIONS
Preventive Visits and Screening Tests

Routine preventive measures refer to a series of regular screenings, checkups, and lifestyle changes that you can undergo to help prevent chronic health problems and to reduce the chance of developing complications from diabetes in the future.

▶ WHAT YOU NEED TO KNOW

There are several routine preventive measures that you can start today:

- **Healthy Diet** A balanced diet can improve blood glucose levels and reduce your risk of heart disease, cancer, and other diseases.
- **Exercise** Regular physical activity can improve blood glucose levels and increase energy, bolster your mood, and improve your overall sense of well-being.
- **Achieve a Healthy Weight** If you are overweight or obese, work with your health care providers to set healthy weight-loss goals.
- **Stop Smoking** Many options are available to help you quit; talk to your provider to find out more.
- **Test Your Blood Glucose at Home** Health care providers recommend testing at least three to four times a day if you have type 1 diabetes. Persons with type 2 diabetes should talk to their provider about how frequently to check; usually, at least once-daily testing (often before breakfast) is recommended.
- **Vaccines** People with diabetes are more likely than others to have serious complications from the flu and require yearly injectable flu shots (preferred over the nasal vaccine for people with diabetes). Other vaccinations, such as the pneumococcal vaccine; the hepatitis B vaccine; the shingles vaccine; and the tetanus, diphtheria, and whooping cough (DTaP) vaccine, are also important (see "Recommended Vaccinations for People with Diabetes" on page 48).
- **Yearly Eye Exam** Patients with diabetes need to be checked with a dilated eye exam yearly to detect complications, such as diabetic retinopathy, so they can be treated in a timely manner.
- **Take Recommended Medications for Blood Pressure** Controlling blood pressure can reduce your chances of developing heart disease.
- **Have Your Cholesterol Checked Regularly** Ask your provider if medications can help prevent the complications of high cholesterol.
- **Aspirin Therapy** Many persons with diabetes benefit from aspirin therapy; talk to your health care provider to see if you are one of them.

Table 3.2. Checklist for routine preventive care in diabetes

PROCEDURE	HOW OFTEN?	TYPICAL GOAL
Hemoglobin A1C	Every 3 months for most people with diabetes; health care providers might space out to every 6 months if results are at goal	Less than 7% (53 mmol/mol) for most nonpregnant adults; sometimes higher (less than 8% or 8.5% or 64 to 69 mmol/mol) for people who are older and have multiple health conditions
Blood pressure check	At every appointment	Less than 140/90 mmHg; sometimes less than 130/80 mmHg for those at high risk of cardiovascular disease
Evaluate your risk of heart disease	At every appointment	Modify lifestyle and other risk factors to prevent disease
Assessment for symptoms of depression	Usually at least yearly	Identify and treat signs of depression if present
Dental cleanings	Twice a year	Maintain oral hygiene, prevent cavities, and identify signs of early dental disease
Cholesterol screen	Usually at least yearly for people above the age of 40	Many persons with diabetes benefit from treatment with statins (especially if above the age of 40) even without high cholesterol levels, given additional cardiovascular protection benefits
Eye exam	Usually yearly but more frequent if signs of eye disease are present	Identify and treat diabetic eye disease as early as possible
Foot exam	At every visit look at feet; a more detailed foot exam will be done yearly	Watch for signs of open ulcerations or injury

Nerve exam (also known as a neuropathy evaluation)	Yearly	Identify if feet have lost the ability to feel touch, vibration, position sense, or temperature
Urine microalbumin (protein) test	Yearly	Identify and treat diabetic kidney disease as early as possible
Serum creatinine	Yearly; sometimes more often	Identify and treat diabetic kidney disease as early as possible
Cancer screening	As recommended by the health care provider based on age	Identify and treat cancer as early as possible

Note: mmHg = millimeters of mercury, used to measure blood pressure.

- **Ask about Cancer Screenings** Find out how often you should be screened for various types of cancer.

Scheduling a Checkup

Persons with diabetes need to visit their health care provider every 3 to 6 months for a routine checkup. This can be spaced out longer if your disease is well controlled. Follow the simple guide outlined in table 3.2 to keep track of the recommended tests and screenings for all persons with diabetes.

WHAT DOES IT ALL MEAN?

- Persons with diabetes can undertake a number of routine preventive measures to prevent complications of diabetes.
- Ask your health care provider which screening tests will be beneficial to you and how frequently they need to be performed.
- Visiting the dentist and eye doctor regularly as recommended, as well as obtaining specialist care if needed for the treatment of diabetic complications such as kidney disease, nerve disease, or heart disease, are key to preventing future health problems.

Recommended Vaccinations for People with Diabetes

A vaccination is the injection of a killed or weakened infectious agent to prevent future infection by the disease-causing agent. Vaccines can be given by mouth, injected, or taken by nose. They trigger the body's immune system to recognize the biological product as foreign, destroy it, and produce antibodies (proteins) that can recognize and destroy any infecting organisms encountered in the future. Though vaccines might not always be on your list of items to discuss at your next appointment, an up-to-date vaccine record is important.

Why? Having diabetes means you're more likely than other people to become ill from common infections that can spread throughout your school, workplace, or community. Frequent handwashing can help prevent illness, to a certain extent, but keeping up with your vaccines is an easy thing you can do to protect your health.

▶ WHAT YOU NEED TO KNOW

Every year, many persons with diabetes die from pneumonia—a dangerous but potentially preventable lung infection. Others succumb to the flu, an infection caused by the influenza virus, which can have serious complications in people with diabetes.

The good news? Both these illnesses can potentially be prevented with vaccines. The bad news? Many people with diabetes remain unprotected. Make a note to ask your health care provider about the following vaccines at your next visit.

Influenza Vaccine
- Recommended for all persons with diabetes, regardless of age (including children 6 months and older).
- Persons with diabetes need a new flu vaccine every year.
- Flu vaccines are available every year, usually beginning around October.
- Two types of influenza vaccines have been available in the past, but only one type is recommended for persons with diabetes, according to the Centers for Disease Control and Prevention (CDC).
- Persons with diabetes should get the flu shot, which is made using an inactive (not live) form of influenza.
- According to the CDC, persons with diabetes should use caution if considering the nasal vaccine, which is made from a weakened form of the live influenza virus and is less preferred. Of note, the availability of the nasal flu vaccine varies from year to year, and the CDC did not recommend

its use for the general population in either the 2016–2017 or 2017–2018 influenza seasons.
- The flu shot may have side effects, including a low-grade fever and transient body aches.

Pneumococcal Vaccine
- Currently, two types of pneumococcal vaccines are available, PPSV23 (sometimes called *pneumovax*) and PCV13 (sometimes called *prevnar*).
- These vaccines can protect against pneumonia caused by different types of pneumococcal bacteria.
- Many people are given a pneumococcal vaccine at the time they are diagnosed with diabetes.
- If you first get the pneumococcal vaccine before your 65th birthday, you will need another shot after you turn 65. In some cases, people will have to wait a few years after their 65th birthday to make sure at least 5 years have passed since their first shot. For example, if you get the pneumococcal vaccine at age 63, you will need a second shot at age 68. Why? Because you are both older than 65 and more than 5 years have passed since your first shot.

Hepatitis B Vaccine
- Recommended for all persons with diabetes from ages 19 to 59 and may be considered for those older than 60 years of age.
- This vaccine is given as a series of three injections spread out over a number of months.

WHAT DOES IT ALL MEAN?
People with diabetes are at higher risk for certain infections. Being up to date with vaccinations is an easy way for a person with diabetes to prevent illness. Talk to your provider about vaccines for the flu, pneumonia, and hepatitis B. Other vaccines routinely given to most other people, such as shingles, tetanus, diphtheria, and whooping cough, are also important to keep up to date.

Special Considerations during Sick Days
Acute illnesses are sicknesses that tend to happen suddenly and unexpectedly. It's best to learn how to prevent the complications that might occur after being sick with viral or bacterial infections, accidental injuries, heart attack, stroke,

or even alcohol abuse. The management of diabetes at home or in the clinical setting may need to be adjusted.

▶ WHAT YOU NEED TO KNOW

Blood glucose levels can rise or fall to dangerous levels during illnesses and other stressful events. For example, people who lose their appetite due to a stomach virus or the seasonal flu might forget to eat, resulting in their blood glucose falling. Low blood glucose can also result from infections or illnesses that affect the kidneys or liver and prolong the effect of diabetes medications (these organs clear some medications from the body). High blood glucose, on the other hand, can result from a variety of factors, including dehydration, missed doses of insulin, medications or drinks that contain added sweeteners, or the body's release of stress hormones in response to illness. Extremely high blood glucose can lead to DKA or hyperglycemic coma—both potentially life-threatening conditions—so it is important to be prepared.

Feeling under the Weather?

- **Alert your Provider** Because people with diabetes are more likely than others to require hospitalization, alert your provider sooner rather than later if you have an acute illness. Be aware that the provider might prescribe a low dose of insulin (or adjust your regular dose of diabetes medications) to regulate blood glucose levels for a short period of time.
- **Consult a Pharmacist** Before buying any over-the-counter medication or filling a prescription, ask a provider or pharmacist if the drug is safe for persons with diabetes. Many medications, including some antibiotics and cold remedies, contain sweeteners and other ingredients that can affect blood glucose levels.
- **Monitor Blood Glucose Frequently** Health care providers may recommend monitoring blood glucose levels more often during an acute illness. People with type 1 diabetes or people with type 2 diabetes on insulin therapy may need to adjust their doses as needed, either up or down, to maintain healthy blood glucose levels.
- **Drink Plenty of Fluids** Dehydration can raise blood glucose levels, as can drinking too many sugar-sweetened beverages, such as fruit juice or soda. Healthy alternatives include water, unsweetened teas, or sugar-free drinks.
- **Treat Fever, Pain, and Cough** In general, pain-reducing pills that contain acetaminophen (for example, Tylenol) or aspirin (but not in children recovering from a viral infection) are safe methods for controlling fever and help

keep glucose levels in check. Over-the-counter medications that reduce inflammation, such as ibuprofen (for example, Motrin or Advil) are generally safe for pain. Sugar-free cough and cold medications are preferred. Check with your health care provider for the best choices for you.

- **Watch for Warning Signs** Go to an emergency room immediately if the following signs or symptoms develop:
    - Persistent vomiting
    - Inability to keep food or drink down for several hours
    - Confusion
    - Difficulty lowering high blood glucose levels
    - Difficulty staying awake

WHAT DOES IT ALL MEAN?

Acute illnesses can cause problems for people with diabetes. Both low and high blood glucose values can occur. Frequently monitoring your blood glucose and staying in close contact with your provider are important to help adjust your medications and prevent problems when you are sick. Sometimes urine ketone testing at home may be recommended in people with type 1 diabetes who are ill. Often, after the short illness resolves, the usual home diabetes regimen can be resumed.

SOCIAL AND LEGAL ISSUES

Social Support for People with Diabetes

Regardless of age, people with diabetes do best when they're surrounded by a supportive network of family, friends, and neighbors. Studies have shown that people who have others to help when needed are highly motivated to take care of themselves and, as a result, develop fewer complications from diabetes.

► WHAT YOU NEED TO KNOW

Children and Teens

Social support is the key to ensuring the health and well-being of children and teens. Parents and caretakers make many decisions on behalf of their children with diabetes. During these years it's especially important for parents to ask many questions. Open communication with their child's health care team, school nurse, and teachers will create a safe, nurturing environment.

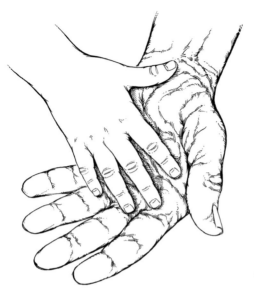

3.3 Having a strong social support network is important for people of any age with diabetes. It helps make diabetes easier to manage. © 2018, Johns Hopkins University, Art as Applied to Medicine

As these children become adolescents, this relationship dynamic changes, but the need for a social network remains stronger than ever. As teens turn more to their friends for support, they take greater ownership of their health. Parents can help by progressively trusting teens with more responsibility and involving them in the decision-making process whenever possible, so they eventually become independent adults who can self-manage their diabetes (figure 3.3).

Adulthood

Though most people with diabetes are fully independent during young adulthood and middle age, family, colleagues, and friends continue to play important roles. They provide healthy outlets for stress relief and support those with diabetes as they work to maintain a healthy lifestyle and treat their disease.

If you're struggling with a desire to eat unhealthy foods, for example, consider inviting friends or neighbors to participate in a healthy meal swap once a week.

Likewise, exercise can become a fun social event by connecting with jogging or walking partners, attending a fitness class, or making a series of appointments with a personal trainer.

The Golden Years

Older adults with diabetes depend on family and caretakers not only for emotional support but for extra reminders sometimes to take medications or for a helpful hand in carrying out their daily routines and making meals.

A person with strong social support can find help when he or she needs it. Help can come from many different sources, including personal relationships, community organizations, diabetes educators or support groups, or online social media networking. This supportive network can make diabetes easier to manage.

If you have diabetes, surround yourself with family and friends who understand your needs and will support your efforts to lead a healthy lifestyle and manage your diabetes. Most providers encourage people with diabetes to bring along family members or friends to clinic visits and keep them actively engaged in their diabetes care.

Driving If You Have Diabetes

The vast majority of people with diabetes drive regularly and safely. Driving by people with diabetes can be safe if the appropriate precautions are taken. Identifying if you're at high risk for having low blood glucose is important. Driving can be impaired by multiple factors, including low blood glucose levels, high blood glucose levels, or diabetes complications.

▶ WHAT YOU NEED TO KNOW

After being diagnosed with diabetes, many people wonder whether they should continue driving to the office or grocery store and are even more concerned about long road trips. The good news is that most people with diabetes are safe drivers—as long as their blood glucose levels are kept in check. Motor vehicle accidents due to diabetes are rare.

What Are the Risks?

While people with diabetes are generally safe on the road, driving can become hazardous when blood glucose levels rise or fall to dangerous levels—*even if the person continues to feel fine.* For this reason, the keys to safety are prevention and preparedness:

- ✓ Always carry a carbohydrate-containing snack in your vehicle in case of low blood glucose (see "Hypoglycemia/Low Blood Glucose" on page 39).
- ✓ Take a blood glucose meter with you in the car, especially if you have a history of low blood glucose levels, in case of an emergency.
- ✓ Remember to test your blood glucose before driving, especially if you have

widely variable blood glucose levels or repeated low blood glucose readings at home.

✓ Don't begin a long drive with low normal blood glucose (that is, 70 to 80 mg/dL) without consuming a carbohydrate, in order to avoid a fall in blood glucose levels while driving.

✓ Stop driving as soon as safely possible at the first sign of low blood glucose (for example, trembling, sweating, irritability, or confusion) and treat the low blood glucose level.

People with type 1 diabetes are at particular risk for sudden, severe drops in blood glucose. These changes can occur with little or no warning and cause confusion, disorientation, and other symptoms that make driving unsafe.

Drivers who are older, are taking insulin, or have had diabetes for more than 10 years with complications such as diabetic eye disease or nerve damage are also at a high risk of having undetected low blood glucose levels. Those who have gone at least 3 years without experiencing confusion or mental status changes due to low blood glucose levels are likely to drive without incident but should still take the appropriate precautions.

Legal Rights

Physicians evaluate each patient individually and make decisions about driving restrictions on a case-by-case basis. Lawmakers must weigh the potential for serious injury against the driver's personal interests when deciding on policies that limit driving. In general, people with insulin-treated diabetes have not often been eligible for interstate commercial driving licenses in the past, or employed by the trucking industry, but diabetes exemptions and waivers are now possible to obtain. Unfortunately, such blanket discrimination sometimes still occurs. Laws change frequently, so contact the motor vehicle administration in your state or the states where you plan to travel to obtain the most up-to-date information.

WHAT DOES IT ALL MEAN?

- Driving safely is not a problem for most people with diabetes.
- Insulin therapy, older age, diabetic eye disease, diabetes nerve damage, and prior episodes of low blood glucose are all risk factors for undetected low blood glucose levels while driving.
- Testing your glucose before you get behind the wheel and carrying a source of carbohydrates in the car can help prevent problems.

- The bottom line: plan ahead and always be prepared, particularly before a long drive.

Employment and Discrimination

People with diabetes may hesitate to discuss their specific needs in the workplace because of fears of discrimination. In this context discrimination refers to the unjust treatment of people because they have diabetes. A casual conversation, a letter from the person's health care provider, or even a copy of this guide can help supervisors understand what diabetes is, how it is treated, and how it can be supported in the workplace.

▶ WHAT YOU NEED TO KNOW

For both employees and supervisors, understanding the difference between myths and facts about diabetes in the workplace can be helpful.

Diabetes in the Workplace: Common Myths

MYTH: People with diabetes are always treated fairly in the workplace.

FACT: People with diabetes are sometimes overlooked for new jobs—or for promotions in their current jobs—because they have a chronic disease. This is known as employment discrimination, and it almost always happens when supervisors are unsure about what diabetes is and how it is treated. This type of discrimination occurs less often as supervisors learn more about diabetes and are educated on its treatment.

MYTH: People with diabetes receive fewer job offers than healthy people.

FACT: During a job search, people are not required to reveal they have diabetes until they've been offered the job. That said, some offers depend on a person's ability to pass a physical exam. If this is the case, the employer and applicant should openly discuss the job duties so they can together determine if any complications of diabetes, such as severe eye disease, might make the work unsafe or unreasonably challenging.

MYTH: Some people with diabetes will be forced to quit their jobs if their supervisors find out they have diabetes.

FACT: It is true that having diabetes can make employment more difficult in a small number of professions without obtaining a waiver or exemption. But the Americans with Disabilities Act requires all other employers to generally support the needs of people with diabetes in the workplace. For example, people with diabetes should be allowed to carry a snack with them and take breaks to self-monitor their blood glucose levels or inject insulin as prescribed by their health care provider.

MYTH: People with diabetes perform poorly at work.

FACT: The truth is that most people with diabetes can be excellent employees. With support from their employers, people with diabetes will succeed in many different types of work, similar to people without diabetes.

MYTH: There is no legal protection for people with diabetes who face discrimination at work.

FACT: Laws against discrimination differ by state and by country. In the United States, the Americans with Disabilities Act protects people with diabetes from unfair treatment in the workplace.

WHAT DOES IT ALL MEAN?

People with diabetes should have the same employment opportunities as other people, and reasonable accommodations should be made to help them treat and manage their blood glucose on the job. Many cases of discrimination may be resolved by educating someone's supervisor about diabetes.

Substance Use in Diabetes

Substance use involves smoking, drinking alcohol, or taking recreational drugs to alter one's mental state. This can interfere with a person's ability to manage his or her diabetes. The use of such substances can also dangerously change blood glucose levels and increase the risk of developing diabetes in people who do not yet have the disease.

▶ WHAT YOU NEED TO KNOW

Substance use is difficult on the body, even for the healthiest of people. But people with diabetes are especially vulnerable to the effects of smoking, alcohol usage, and recreational drug use (table 3.3).

Table 3.3. Effects of using different substances on diabetes management

SMOKING

Cigarette smoking doubles the risk of developing diabetes and increases the risk of heart disease, strokes, circulatory problems in the legs, and many cancers. For those who smoke, stopping cigarettes can greatly help prevent the cardiovascular, eye, kidney, and nerve complications of diabetes from developing. Research has shown that persons with diabetes who stop smoking have improved blood pressure and fewer kidney and nerve complications from diabetes after just 1 year. Programs shown to help smokers stop include telephone quit lines that provide counseling, as well as several medications.

ALCOHOL

Heavy alcohol use—meaning more than four drinks per day—increases the risk of type 2 diabetes. People under the influence of alcohol often don't notice their blood glucose level dropping until it reaches a dangerously low level. Excessive alcohol use can deplete the liver of its glucose stores and prevent it from releasing glucose into the blood when it is needed, such as when blood glucose levels are low (*hypoglycemia*), which can be life-threatening. This can be especially problematic in people with type 1 diabetes or with type 2 diabetes who take insulin.

COCAINE

Regardless of whether cocaine is smoked, snorted, injected, or swallowed, it harms nearly all parts of the body. Cocaine may cause blood glucose levels to skyrocket and can quickly lead to a life-threatening complication called *diabetic ketoacidosis* (see "Diabetic Ketoacidosis" on page 35), which requires hospitalization, sometimes even in persons with type 2 diabetes. In addition, cocaine strains the heart, increasing the risk of heart attack and stroke.

MARIJUANA

Nearly half of all Americans have tried marijuana, or cannabis, at some point in their lives. It remains a commonly used illegal substance, although it has now become legal in some states. Because this drug causes food cravings, people with diabetes may find it hard to control their hunger if they use it. Binge eating can make it much more difficult to control blood glucose levels.

HEROIN

Heroin use may affect the amount of insulin released by the pancreas, but more research is needed. Periods of drowsiness and confusion after heroin use can lead to missed insulin injections or pills for diabetes. This makes it increasingly difficult to manage the condition. Difficult-to-manage diabetes can lead to a range of health complications.

It's important to understand how these substances affect your blood glucose levels—and to avoid them as much as possible. If you can't cut back or quit, ask for help.

How Much Is Too Much?

Chances are, you've filled out paperwork at a health care provider's office that asked how often you drink alcohol, smoke, or use recreational drugs. Your provider uses this information to gauge the impact of these substances on your everyday life. It's important to answer these truthfully. It won't be used to get you in trouble but can help save your life.

If it seems as if substance use is harming your health, your provider might follow up with more detailed questions. For instance, some questions that your provider might ask about drinking alcohol include:

- ✓ Have you ever felt you ought to cut down on your drinking?
- ✓ Have people annoyed you by criticizing your drinking?
- ✓ Have you ever felt guilty about your drinking?
- ✓ Have you ever had a drink first thing in the morning to get rid of a hangover or steady your nerves?

This information can reveal your risk of *substance use disorder*, a medical condition requiring treatment and often rehabilitation.

Why Quit?

People diagnosed with substance use disorder often find it difficult to control how frequently they smoke or the amount of alcohol or recreational drugs they consume. They may find it hard to quit—even when they know their life is at stake.

If you find yourself in this situation, don't be afraid to speak up at your next appointment. Your providers will not get you in trouble but rather will work with you to devise a strategy for quitting that can also help your diabetes.

Your health care provider may set goals that you can work on at home, like avoiding social situations that trigger you to smoke, drink, or use recreational drugs or by cutting down a little bit at a time. Your provider may also recommend a 12-step group, an outpatient or inpatient rehabilitation program, or prescription medicines to help prevent withdrawal symptoms.

WHAT DOES IT ALL MEAN?

Smoking, drinking alcohol, and using recreational drugs, which alter one's mental state, may result in abnormal glucose levels, either by directly affecting glucose or by leading to behaviors that lead to worsening diabetes management. If you feel you might have a substance use problem, let your medical providers know, so they can help you combat the problem and better prevent or manage diabetes.

Preparing for Natural Disasters and Emergencies

Disasters can occur anytime and anywhere. Hurricanes, floods, tornadoes, and terrorism are unpredictable and can disrupt the lives of people with chronic illnesses such as diabetes.

When disaster strikes, communities can be left without access to electricity, shelter, or communication, and this can affect the storage or availability of medications for diabetes. Stressful situations can wreak havoc on your blood glucose levels, while injuries increase the risk of infection. As the disaster unfolds, access to medical care might be limited or unavailable.

▶ WHAT YOU NEED TO KNOW

Follow the steps below to prepare for disaster *before* it strikes. Share these guidelines with your family and friends so that you will be prepared to act quickly and responsibly.

- *Stay on top of your health with good self-care and stress management.* This will help ensure you're as resilient as possible during an emergency situation. Make sure you're up to date on immunizations, including your tetanus shot.
- *Always remember shoes, food, and water.* During emergencies, wear sturdy shoes and check your feet daily for cuts, sores, or signs of infection, such as red, hot, or puffy skin—especially if you have nerve damage. Drink plenty of clean water and maintain a healthy diet. Seek emergency care as soon as possible if you become tired, feel weak, or develop a fever or stomach cramps.
- *Shelter in place, if possible.* It's important to stock your home with ample food, medicines, and supplies so that you can avoid going to a shelter, where there may be limited healthy foods, cramped sleeping spaces, and reduced access to prescription medicines and toiletries. If your community is ordered to evacuate, do so as quickly as possible.
- *Make a waterproof disaster "Go Kit."* Be prepared to leave your home at a moment's notice, especially if you anticipate an evacuation in the near future. Pack a duffel bag ahead of time with everything needed to manage your diabetes for a few days. Here are a few "must-have" items:

✓ Paper copies of your medical history and prescriptions, contact info for your physician and family, names of medications and doses, recent lab results, allergies, and blood type. Keep hotline numbers for national diabetes associations handy. Place in a plastic storage bag.

✓ Enough glucose test strips and lancets to last several days

✓ Blood glucose meter, test strips, lancets, and extra batteries

✓ Medications, including insulin, and insulin pump supplies

✓ Extra syringes and needles

✓ Glucose tabs or gels

✓ Antibiotic ointments/creams

✓ Glucagon emergency kits

✓ Plenty of healthy prepackaged snacks, such as peanut butter, powdered milk, unsweetened cereal, cans of tuna and chicken, nuts, and cheese crackers

- *Keep your insulin stored at the proper temperature.* Storing your insulin at the correct temperature is the key to making sure it works well during a disaster, especially during the hot summer months. If you need to switch to a different type of insulin during an emergency, ask a health care provider for help. Do not do this without help, as many insulin types are available, and they are not all the same.

  − *If you have access to a refrigerator*:
    ○ Store extra insulin, including pens, in the refrigerator until their expiration date.
    ○ Once opened or in use, discard insulin after 28 days. Open insulin vials or pens can be kept at room temperature or in the refrigerator depending on the insulin type.

  − *If you do not have access to a refrigerator*:
    ○ Insulin vials or cartridges that have *not* been opened can be kept at room temperature (ranges between 59 to 86 degrees Fahrenheit) for up to 28 or 42 days depending on the insulin type as long as the storage area is not extremely hot or cold.
    ○ Insulin pens will last at room temperature (ranges between 59 to 86 degrees Fahrenheit) for a few weeks, depending on the type:
      − NPH insulin pens will last for 14 days.
      − Insulin lispro, aspart, glulisine, and glargine U-100 pens will last for 28 days.
      − Insulin detemir and insulin glargine U-300 pens will last for 42 days.
      − Insulin degludec pens will last for 56 days.

WHAT DOES IT ALL MEAN?

Natural disasters or terrorist events are unpredictable. Preparing an emergency kit with medicines and supplies is crucial should an event occur. Special attention needs to be taken if you use insulin. Specifically, having an extra supply of insulin and knowing how to store it can help in times of emergency.

Chapter 4

DIABETES IN SPECIAL POPULATIONS

Children and Type 2 Diabetes

Given the rising rates of obesity, type 2 diabetes is unfortunately no longer just a disease of adults. Children, particularly those from racial or ethnic minority groups, are also at risk for developing type 2 diabetes. A healthy lifestyle, including a diet and exercise that avoids obesity, is key to preventing type 2 diabetes in children.

▶ WHAT YOU NEED TO KNOW

Is Adult-Onset Diabetes the Same as Type 2 Diabetes?

In the past, type 2 diabetes was called *adult-onset* diabetes. Over the past few decades, type 2 diabetes has become more common in children, related in part to rising obesity rates. Conversely, type 1 diabetes is also sometimes diagnosed in adulthood. For this reason, *type 2 diabetes* is the preferred term to refer to diabetes related to insulin resistance and obesity.

What Is the Difference between Type 2 Diabetes in Adults versus Children?

The disease is generally similar in adults and children. In both cases, the muscles and other organs in the body, such as the liver, stop responding normally to insulin, forcing the pancreas to work harder to produce enough insulin to maintain normal blood glucose levels. Excess body fat makes it more difficult for the body to appropriately respond to insulin and maintain blood glucose levels in a healthy range.

At What Age Does Type 2 Diabetes Develop?

Type 2 diabetes is most commonly diagnosed in adults during midlife. It is relatively less common in children younger than 10 years who have not yet reached puberty. The disease is becoming more common in children aged 10 years and older or after puberty.

Which Symptoms Develop in Children?

Like adults with type 2 diabetes, children with the disease will often complain that they're thirstier than usual. They might urinate a lot or unexpectedly lose weight (see "Differences between Type 1 and Type 2 Diabetes" on page 15). Unlike adults, children with type 2 diabetes may also develop diabetic ketoacidosis (see "Diabetic Ketoacidosis" on page 35), a dangerous condition that occurs with severely high blood glucose levels and the buildup of acid in the blood. These children have a few days of nausea and vomiting that progresses to confusion and lethargy.

How Is Type 2 Diabetes Diagnosed in Children?

Overweight or obese children who have family members with diabetes or other risk factors for diabetes may be screened by their health care providers (see "Risk Factors for Type 2 Diabetes" on page 13). Also, because type 2 diabetes is more common in nonwhite populations (that is, blacks, Hispanics, and Asians), overweight and obese children from ethnic minority populations should be screened for diabetes if they are at higher risk (figure 4.1). Testing similar to that for adults is also used for children: hemoglobin A1C, fasting plasma glucose, or an oral glucose tolerance test (see "Diagnosing Diabetes" on page 11).

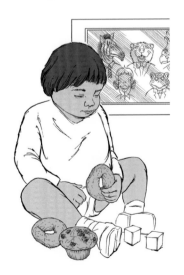

4.1 Increased rates of obesity have led to a rise in childhood type 2 diabetes. A healthy diet, regular physical activity, and weight loss can help prevent diabetes in children. © 2018, Johns Hopkins University, Art as Applied to Medicine

Are There Any Child-Friendly Treatments for Type 2 Diabetes?

An important part of treatment will generally be a recommendation for a healthy diet and regular exercise. Often, children with diabetes work closely with dietitians to devise a plan for healthy eating and for weight loss if the child is overweight or obese. In addition, the child with type 2 diabetes will generally be prescribed an oral pill called *metformin* (see "Metformin" on page 225). Children who have more severe diabetes—those with A1C levels higher than 8.5% or 69 millimoles per mole (mmol/mol)—are usually also started on daily insulin injections. Any child with type 2 diabetes who develops ketoacidosis will have to be treated with daily insulin injections. The goal of treatment is to reduce the child's A1C level to a range considered healthy by the patient's provider. This range will differ for each child, but most children and adolescents with diabetes try to reduce their level to less than 7% to 7.5% (53 to 58 mmol/mol).

What Routine Appointments Should I Schedule for My Child with Type 2 Diabetes?

- **Every 3 to 6 Months** Measure A1C level, lipids, and other routine blood tests as needed; check blood pressure with a regular physical exam by a diabetes provider.
- **Every Year or Every Few Years** Vaccinations as recommended. The frequency of some routine preventive measures (see "Recommended Vaccinations for People with Diabetes" on page 48) will be similar to that of adults while others will be different; check with your health care provider.

How Can Type 2 Diabetes in Children Be Prevented?

Children who are overweight or obese are at risk of developing type 2 diabetes. Weight loss, healthy eating habits, and regular exercise are key to preventing this disease.

What Else Should a Child with Type 2 Diabetes Do for His or Her Health?

Type 2 diabetes increases the risk of developing heart disease or having a stroke. While these complications would usually not occur until adulthood, it is very important that a child with type 2 diabetes does not start smoking (or stops smoking if they already do). Starting at puberty, education on pregnancy prevention is critical.

WHAT DOES IT ALL MEAN?

Type 2 diabetes is no longer just a disease for adults. The increasing rate of childhood obesity combined with a lack of exercise has led to a rise in type 2 diabetes among children. Having parents with type 2 diabetes or belonging to a racial or ethnic minority group further increases a child's risk. Along with medication, focusing on increased activity, dietary changes, and weight loss as appropriate is crucial in the treatment of type 2 diabetes for children.

Older Adults and Diabetes

As we get older, our bodies change in ways that may make diabetes more likely to occur. Exercise may become less frequent. Weight changes can occur. Hormones change. All these factors can add up to an increased risk of diabetes. People with diabetes are also living longer. A growing number of people with diabetes are age 65 years and older, and the treatment of diabetes may represent unique challenges in older adults.

▶ WHAT YOU NEED TO KNOW

One in four persons who are 65 years and older have diabetes. Together, diabetes and prediabetes affected nearly three-quarters of older adults in 2017. Medicare now provides coverage to all older adults with prediabetes who wish to enroll in a yearlong Diabetes Prevention Program (see "Landmark Studies in Diabetes Care" on page 6) that focuses on intensive lifestyle changes to delay the progression to diabetes.

Older people with diabetes experience many of the same symptoms that affect younger patients:

- Unusual thirstiness
- Urinating often
- Weight loss
- Blurry vision

Caring for the Older Person with Diabetes

Memory problems or other health issues can make it more difficult for the older adult to manage his or her diabetes (figure 4.2). Here are a few common issues that arise:

- Poor vision can make it difficult for older people with diabetes to check their own blood glucose or draw up and administer the right amount of insulin.
- Low blood glucose levels are more common in older persons, particularly among those on multiple medications, and can be dangerous.
- Depression and memory problems may occur in older persons with diabe-

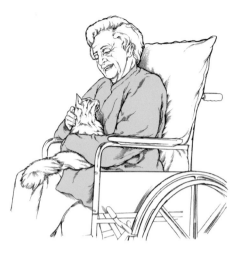

4.2 Prediabetes and diabetes are common in older adults. This population faces unique challenges related to aging that can potentially make diabetes more complicated to manage. © 2018, Johns Hopkins University, Art as Applied to Medicine

tes, making it less likely they will remember to monitor their blood glucose at home, take their medications, watch their diet, and self-manage their disease.

- Moving around and performing daily activities, such as preparing meals, shopping, and cleaning the house, can prove especially challenging when an older person has diabetes because of weaker muscles and difficulty with walking.
- Injuries or fractures from accidental falls are common in older patients with diabetes due to complications such as nerve damage, low blood glucose, and vision loss.
- Difficulty controlling and holding urine, a condition called *incontinence*, often affects older adults with very high glucose levels or nerve damage.

Healthy Goals

Lifestyle changes are imperative in older persons with diabetes, just as for younger persons:

- **Physical Activity** Get outdoors—gardening or taking daily walks around a park, neighborhood, or shopping mall are easy ways to incorporate physical activity into your daily routine. Muscle-strengthening exercises (for example, lifting weights) are also particularly important in the older person with diabetes. Check with your health care provider first before starting a new exercise regimen.
- **Eat a Healthy Diet** Ask your health care provider to recommend a dietitian who can help you create a nutritious meal plan. If you are overweight or obese, ask your health care provider if weight loss can help.

When healthy lifestyle changes aren't enough, your health care provider might prescribe pills or insulin to keep your blood glucose levels under control. Medication treatment is often based on the A1C test, which reveals how well-controlled blood glucose levels have been for the past 3 months. Health care providers prefer to set individual treatment goals with older adults to reduce the risk of complications, minimize low blood glucose levels, and optimize quality of life. In general, most medications that can be used in younger persons with diabetes can be safely used in older persons, as well. However, older persons may be more likely to experience low blood glucose levels. Medications that stimulate insulin production (such as sulfonylureas or meglitinides) or insulin therapy itself may sometimes need to be carefully dosed to prevent hypoglycemia.

What Is Your A1C Goal?

Reasonable goals for people with diabetes are included in table 4.1.

Table 4.1. Commonly recommended A1C goals in older adults

POPULATION	A1C GOAL
People who are not pregnant and <65 years of age	Less than 7% (53 mmol/mol)
Older people (65 years and older) with no other major health concerns who are otherwise healthy	Less than 7%–7.5% (53 to 58 mmol/mol)
Older people (65 years and older) who have multiple other medical conditions, limited physical functioning, or repeated low blood glucose levels	Less than 8%–8.5% (64 to 69 mmol/mol), depending on other medical conditions

WHAT DOES IT ALL MEAN?

- Diabetes in older persons is a huge public health concern.
- Prediabetes is also common and represents an opportunity for targeted prevention efforts in older adults.
- Older adults may face many unique challenges in their everyday lives that can make it difficult to manage their diabetes. Health care providers prefer to set

individual treatment goals with each person based on his or her overall health status and other factors.

Diabetes among People Living with HIV

Human immunodeficiency virus (HIV) is the virus that causes acquired immune deficiency syndrome (AIDS). People with HIV or AIDS have a compromised immune system and are more likely than other people to catch the common cold, develop bacterial infections, or acquire a number of other serious illnesses. People with HIV are also at a higher risk of developing diabetes from traditional risk factors, the virus itself, and from the medicines used to treat the virus.

▶ WHAT YOU NEED TO KNOW

People with HIV are treated with drugs called *antiretrovirals* that prevent the virus from growing inside the body. With these drugs, people with HIV enjoy longer and healthier lives now than they did just 20 years ago. Like most drugs, however, they can have undesirable side effects. In particular, some antiretrovirals can change the body's response to insulin and make the body resistant to its effects, which sometimes leads to diabetes. First-generation antiretroviral drugs, such as stavudine and indinavir, which have now largely decreased in use, have been strongly associated with developing diabetes. However, newer agents for HIV might also be associated with the development of diabetes.

*How Does Diabetes among People with HIV Differ
from Other Types?*

In the past, diabetes was often related to the drugs used to treat HIV rather than to the typical diabetes risk factors alone. Diabetes is much more common in people with HIV taking antiretroviral medications (particularly older versions). Other conditions, such as hepatitis C or low testosterone levels, are more common in people with HIV and may also contribute to a higher risk of diabetes. Nonetheless, people with HIV are still more likely to develop diabetes if they have the traditional risk factors and are overweight, lack physical activity, have increased abdominal fat, have a family history of diabetes, are older, or belong to a racial or ethnic minority group. Some people with HIV may be asked to have their blood glucose levels checked before and for a few months after starting HIV medicines.

What Health Complications Can Occur in People with HIV Who Have Diabetes?

People with HIV who have diabetes are at risk for complications from both HIV and diabetes. These people have an especially high risk of developing kidney disease, and they are twice as likely as others to develop heart disease.

How Is Diabetes among People with HIV Diagnosed and Treated?

The same criteria to diagnose other people with diabetes are used for those with HIV. However, the A1C may underestimate average glucose levels in people with HIV. For this reason, testing with fasting plasma glucose is usually preferred. Some guidelines suggest testing for diabetes every 6 to 12 months in all HIV-infected people.

As always, exercise and a healthy diet are key to controlling diabetes. Lifestyle factors and preventive strategies include the following:

- Stop smoking.
- Lose weight.
- Control your blood pressure and cholesterol.
- Avoid illegal drugs.
- Ask your health care provider about aspirin therapy, which may be appropriate for some people with HIV and diabetes.

If lifestyle changes aren't enough to keep blood glucose within healthy limits, the health care provider might suggest switching to other therapies for HIV that are less likely to raise blood glucose levels. If diabetes medications are needed, metformin is considered a first-line therapy, and the decision regarding other therapies needs to be individualized. If the pills are ineffective or interact with HIV medications, the provider might consider insulin therapy.

How Often Should Those with HIV and Diabetes Visit Their Physician?

Like people without HIV, those with HIV and diabetes should visit their provider for regular checkups and to measure their hemoglobin A1C levels. In between appointments, people on diabetes medications may be asked to monitor their blood glucose regularly.

WHAT DOES IT ALL MEAN?

- People with HIV are more likely to develop diabetes than other people.
- People with HIV who have diabetes have a higher risk of complications compared to people who only have HIV and those who only have diabetes.

- A healthy lifestyle can go a long way toward controlling blood glucose and preventing future complications.

Race and Ethnic Disparities in Diabetes

Health disparities refer to preventable differences in the complications from diseases such as diabetes. Race or ethnic health disparities can result in greater obstacles to health based on a person's racial or ethnic group.

▶ WHAT YOU NEED TO KNOW

Diabetes has become increasingly common, affecting more than 400 million people worldwide. The number of people with diabetes is expected to continue rising dramatically as the world's population increasingly shifts to an unhealthy diet and sedentary lifestyle. The impact will be greatest in low- and middle-income countries. The condition is especially common in China, India, the Middle East, and northern Africa.

Approximately one-third of the U.S. population identifies themselves as belonging to a racial or ethnic minority population. Diabetes is more common in some ethnic groups than others—especially groups that have a higher rate of obesity. African Americans are almost twice as likely to have type 2 diabetes than non-Hispanic whites and are also more likely to have diabetic complications, such as kidney disease, blindness, and amputations. Other ethnic groups at higher risk of diabetes include American Indians, Hispanics and Latinos, Asian Americans, and Pacific Islanders.

Some ethnic groups are also more likely to have high blood pressure or high cholesterol, which can contribute to a higher rate of diabetes complications. Asian Americans have a greater percentage of body fat compared to people of other ethnicities with the same body weight. A body mass index of 23 kilograms per square meter or greater is considered overweight in Asian Americans. Reducing racial or ethnic disparities can help dramatically dampen the rising epidemic of diabetes in the United States and worldwide.

Equal Access

Everyone—regardless of skin color or cultural practice—has a right to quality health care. Unfortunately, persons of minority populations may face greater obstacles to accessing health care. African Americans and American Indians are twice as likely to die from diabetes compared to non-Hispanic whites with diabetes. This may be related to poverty, crime, lack of access to healthy foods and health care clinics, and cultural attitudes or behaviors that can affect diabetes management. Limited access to high-quality education, safe housing, affordable public transportation, health insurance, clean water and nonpolluted air, and culturally sensitive health care providers also contribute to health disparities.

How Can I Help?

Look around your community for organizations that bring together people with diabetes from diverse backgrounds with representatives from health care organizations, the community, health care systems, and health care providers.

Other organizations are working to improve basic living conditions so that neighborhoods are safer, greener, and more accessible to medical services. This can help reduce stress, encourage physical activity and healthy diets, and limit the effects of poverty and violence for persons of all racial and ethnic backgrounds. Consider volunteering or donating to these organizations.

WHAT DOES IT ALL MEAN?

If you belong to an ethnic minority population, you may be more likely to develop diabetes and related complications. While everyone should have equal access to good-quality health care, unfortunately, this is not always the case. In addition to race or ethnicity, there may be disparities by age, sex, sexual orientation, disability, socioeconomic status, and geographic location that prevent optimal health. Talk to your health care provider about resources that may be available in your community to reduce these disparities and improve health outcomes for all people with diabetes.

Diabetes in American Indians

Hundreds of tribal communities—each with distinct cultures, traditions, and languages—are collectively known as Native Americans in the United States and as the First Nations in Canada. Diabetes is more common in these tribal communities than the rest of population.

▶ WHAT YOU NEED TO KNOW

Diabetes rates are rising rapidly, especially among children and teens. Diabetes is more than twice as common among American Indians than the general population. American Indians also have higher rates of medical conditions related to diabetes, including cancer. This is due to a number of reasons, including fewer quality supermarkets, a lack of designated exercise areas, and less accessibility to health care in tribal communities. American Indians also have high obesity rates, partly due to the widespread adoption of a Western diet rich in high-fat, processed foods.

TIPS FOR PERSONS WITH DIABETES IN TRIBAL COMMUNITIES

- Replace processed foods with traditional, home-cooked foods and low-sugar drinks. Many healthy meals can be prepared using foods bought with food stamps or the Women, Infants, and Children (WIC) nutrition program.
- Keep portion sizes moderate and read nutrition labels for serving sizes.
- Reduce alcohol consumption to keep blood glucose levels stable.
- Get up and exercise but start slowly, especially if you have never exercised before.
- Organize community fitness competitions using pedometers.
- Record your goals and achievements using pen and paper or smartphone apps.
- Follow up with a health professional to make sure you're on track.
- Start slow, but making steady gains can add up to much better health.

TIPS TO SHARE WITH YOUR HEALTH CARE PROVIDER IN TRIBAL COMMUNITIES

- Providers may need to deliver diabetes education in a way that speaks to the community's unique culture, such as by demonstrating how traditional foods, tribal healing practices, and community elders can help build healthy lifestyles.
- Providers should also recognize cultural beliefs that may undermine health (such as the idea that larger body sizes are healthier in some cultures) and empower community members to take charge of their health.
- Improved access is needed for the resources available through the U.S. Special Diabetes Program for Indians, Indian Health Services, community wellness centers, and schools.
- Helping communities access and afford healthy foods can promote effective lifestyle changes.

WHAT DOES IT ALL MEAN?

American Indians have high rates of obesity and diabetes. Addressing cultural practices and belief systems, as well as providing community programs that increase access to healthy supermarkets and facilities to exercise, are uniquely important to managing diabetes in this population.

Diabetes Care during Times of Religious Fasting

The practice of *fasting*, or avoiding food for a certain period, is a cleansing ritual for many cultures and religions. Many people with diabetes belong to the Islamic faith around the world and regularly fast for Ramadan. As you might imagine, certain safeguards are needed to protect blood glucose levels during this spiritual practice.

▶ **WHAT YOU NEED TO KNOW**

Fasting is common in many cultures and religions. Fasting is one of the five pillars of Islam. Ramadan is an obligatory monthlong fast during the ninth month of the Islamic calendar. This ritual differs from other nonobligatory fasting days that may occur during the year. While fasting is usually mandatory for all Muslim adults, certain groups are exempted, such as pregnant or breastfeeding women and those with serious medical conditions.

During Ramadan, each day before dawn, Muslims observe a prefast meal (*suhoor*). The fasting day starts at dawn and ends at sunset with a meal (*iftar*) that is typically rich in carbohydrates and fats. Fasting may lead to complications in people with diabetes. These complications may arise from the following:

- Skipping medicines during the fast to avoid low blood sugar can lead to dangerously high blood glucose levels.
- Patients who live farther from the equator have longer fasting days during the summer, which can cause blood glucose levels to drop.
- Long days and physical exertion without eating or drinking may increase the stress on the body and lead to dehydration and low blood glucose levels.

Preparing for the Ramadan Fast

Visit your health care provider 1 to 2 months before religious fasting to get an assessment of your overall health and blood glucose levels. The provider will determine your health risks and help you prepare for the fast.

People at *very high risk* of difficulties during fasting include those who have experienced an acute blood glucose crisis requiring hospitalization within 3 months of the religious fast, are on multiple daily injections of insulin, have low or very high blood glucose levels, have advanced heart or kidney disease, or have poorly managed type 1 diabetes. This group also includes pregnant women or people who perform a lot of physical labor.

People at *high risk* of difficulties during fasting are those who have poorly managed type 2 diabetes or well-controlled type 1 diabetes who are taking multiple daily injections of insulin.

People at *moderate or low risk* of difficulties during fasting are those who have well-managed diabetes on oral medication alone or take oral medication and a single daily injection of insulin to control their blood glucose levels.

Monitor your body for signs of distress:

- Know the signs of low or high blood glucose levels.
- Monitor your blood glucose levels and break the fast if they drop below 70 milligrams per deciliter (mg/dL).
- Eat and drink whenever possible but avoid processed sugars and saturated fats.
- Only do hard labor or intense physical activity at the beginning of the day.
- After Ramadan or religious fasting, adjust your medicine dose back to the previous schedule.

Medication Adjustments during Ramadan or Religious Fasting

Depending on whether you are more or less likely to have difficulties during times of religious fasting, your provider may recommend adjustments to your medications for diabetes. Often, medications with a low risk of *hypoglycemia* (low blood glucose levels), such as metformin, are considered safe. Other medications such as sulfonylureas may be discouraged during fasting, given the higher risk of hypoglycemia. It is important to keep hydrated, especially when taking medicines such as SGLT2 inhibitors. While insulin can be safely used, dosing adjustments are often required. If you're taking 70/30 premixed insulin, you may be advised to take the full morning dose in the evening with the large meal that breaks the fast and to take a reduced evening dose with the morning meal. Be sure to ask your provider for specific advice about medication changes that need to be made during times of fasting.

WHAT DOES IT ALL MEAN?

- Fasting is common in many cultures and religions around the world.
- Ramadan is perhaps one of the longest religious fasts, occurring over 1 month every year in the Islam religion.
- Medication changes to prevent dehydration and low (or high) blood glucose levels may be necessary during Ramadan and are usually common during times of fasting in other religions, as well.

Diabetes Care during a Hospital Stay

People with diabetes enter the hospital for a variety of reasons—sometimes for poorly controlled blood glucose levels at home but often for reasons not related to their diabetes. Regardless of the reason for admission, people with diabetes require special care during their hospitalization. They may also need changes to their diabetes medications and special dietary considerations while in the hospital.

▶ WHAT YOU NEED TO KNOW

High blood glucose levels that are left untreated can make your hospital stay longer by

- increasing the risk for infections,
- prolonging the time needed for wounds to heal,
- causing a buildup of acid in the bloodstream (see "Diabetic Ketoacidosis" on page 35),
- causing dehydration and kidney failure, and
- increasing the risk of complications after a solid organ or bone marrow transplant.

However, hypoglycemia can also be dangerous in the hospital. Unfortunately, an unpredictable schedule of diagnostic tests and varying meal times can increase the likelihood of hypoglycemia. Because of this, glucose goals in the hospital are typically less strict than at home. A goal glucose of 140 to 180 mg/dL or 7.8 to 10.0 millimoles per liter (mmol/L) is appropriate for most hospitalized patients.

The hospital health care provider will tailor your care to keep blood glucose at safe levels. This is a challenging task because many common hospital procedures can complicate blood glucose management (see table 4.2).

To work around these challenges, the hospital provider might make temporary changes to the daily medication regimen. Many people with diabetes are able to return to their regular regimen after leaving the hospital if they were previously well managed, but more often, some dose changes are made.

Medication Changes

To prevent hypoglycemia or other side effects, particularly after certain hospital tests, oral diabetes medications (for example, metformin) might not be given during the hospital stay.

Instead, many people with long-standing diabetes are given insulin (even those not previously on it). In the hospital, giving insulin is often preferred and can be adjusted based on changing dietary regimens and hospital procedures.

People with newly diagnosed type 2 diabetes or high blood glucose levels

Table 4.2. Procedures in the hospital that can affect diabetes management

MAY LOWER BLOOD GLUCOSE LEVELS	MAY RAISE BLOOD GLUCOSE LEVELS
"Nothing by mouth" orders (NPO)	Tube feedings
Poor appetite	Intravenous nutrition
Specific medications (for example, antibiotics)	Some dextrose-containing intravenous fluids or medications
Late meals	Specific medications that may raise blood glucose levels (for example, steroids)

may be given insulin to maintain their blood glucose at healthy levels. Often these people can be converted to oral medications by the time of discharge if they are only using small doses of insulin in the hospital.

Special Help for Insulin Pumps

For those with insulin pumps, hospital factors such as stress, pain, medication, or mental distractions can make it difficult to keep track of things during a hospital stay.

However, many people with diabetes using insulin pumps can still safely use these devices while in the hospital. Nurses can help monitor pump use and double-check the medical record to ensure an accurate dosing schedule. In some circumstances, people with diabetes may be advised not to use their insulin pump in the hospital for safety reasons. These people will receive multiple daily insulin injections instead and can often resume using their insulin pump when discharged under guidance from the health care team.

A guide for calculating the correct doses of basal and nutritional insulin is shown in box 4.1.

Nutrition and Diet

At home, rapid-acting mealtime insulin is usually taken immediately prior to a meal. In the hospital, people may eat less than expected, so it is sometimes safer to give the mealtime insulin right after a meal and make dose adjustments based on how much is eaten.

People with diabetes preparing for surgery or other procedures may not be allowed to eat or drink. In such cases, the provider may recommend decreasing the level of basal (intermediate- or long-acting) insulin moderately. Mealtime insulin is held until meals start again, but correctional insulin is continued to bring down high blood glucose levels.

Going Home

Before leaving the hospital, it is important to discuss any medication changes and create a plan for home-based care.

People with diabetes should continue monitoring their blood glucose levels at home and contact their health care provider if these levels are too high or low (box 4.2). The home glucose meter and blood glucose log should be taken to the next follow-up appointment, which usually occurs a few weeks after leaving the hospital. Sometimes, additional medication changes will need to be made.

- Often, medications change when a person with diabetes is admitted to a hospital. For instance, metformin is often held back.
- Some medications, such as steroids, may increase blood glucose readings in the hospital and require the adjustment of insulin doses (see "Steroid-Induced Diabetes" on page 28).
- Insulin therapy is often preferred to oral medications in the hospital.
- People with diabetes should generally receive carbohydrate-controlled diets in the hospital unless there are other considerations.
- Glucose goals may be different when hospitalized compared to glucose goals at home. Often, people with diabetes can return to their home medication regimen upon discharge if they were previously well managed.
- A diabetes management service (including a physician, nurse practitioner, diabetes educator, and possibly a dietitian) may be available in the hospital to help with difficult-to-manage diabetes.
- On discharge, it is important to understand any changes to the diabetes regimen and when to contact a health care provider.

Chapter 5

LIFESTYLE AND BEHAVIORAL CHANGES IN DIABETES

DIABETES EDUCATION
Overcoming Denial, Fear, and Other Obstacles to Good Health

A diagnosis of diabetes can be overwhelming and carries with it many different emotions. It requires understanding a new and complex disease. Adjusting diet and exercise, taking new medications, and checking finger-stick blood glucose readings are all changes that usually need to happen. It is important to recognize any potential difficulties and find ways to overcome them.

► WHAT YOU NEED TO KNOW

A diagnosis of diabetes often requires major lifestyle changes to your routine. But it's important to remember that you're not alone! Even if diabetes is new territory to you, chances are that your health care provider has seen it all. Sharing your concerns is a great way to get help. Some of the common obstacles people face with diabetes—and their possible solutions—are described in this chapter.

Styles of Learning

There's much to learn about diabetes management, so don't be hesitant to ask questions if you have trouble understanding what your health care provider tells you during the clinic visit. Some people learn better when they watch videos, while others prefer to read articles or brochures or attend classes. If you want to find out about different learning tools, speak up. Many types of diabetes education resources exist, and your health care provider may have a trick that can help you understand all that you need to know. Find the method that works best for you.

Cultural Practices

All cultures embrace different practices, including alternative medicines, dietary restrictions, health beliefs, and spiritual customs. These may result in your health care provider adjusting the approach to your diabetes management. Be sure to tell your providers about these practices, so they can help you achieve and maintain good health.

Disabilities

People with poor vision often find it helpful to use voice-activated or large-print glucose meters with a bright backlight. If you're hard of hearing, your provider may provide written material or computer-assisted learning devices.

People who have trouble with arthritis or manipulating their hands may need extra help when it comes to insulin shots and blood glucose meters. Ask your provider to help you learn simple techniques for using your blood glucose meter. Many people with physical disabilities find it less cumbersome to use insulin pens or prefilled syringes. Tell your providers about these difficulties so they can help.

Emotional Care

Not uncommonly, people with diabetes feel shocked, angry, or upset when they first learn they have diabetes or when they encounter setbacks after living with the disease for many years. As many as one-third of people with diabetes are diagnosed with depression (see "Depression" on page 110). If you notice these feelings, talk about them with your provider and consider seeing a mental health counselor. Depression can get in the way of your self-care, so it's important to address these emotions with your diabetes care provider or therapist. Consider doing a quiet reflective practice, such as meditation (see "Meditation and Stress Reduction" on page 266), or other activities that help your mood and reduce stress.

Perseverance

If you develop complications of diabetes, don't feel discouraged. Diabetes tends to get worse, and complications develop, with a longer duration of the disease. Complications may arise despite your best efforts at healthy living. Don't get disheartened because continued good self-management can help slow down these and future complications.

Pricking Fingers for Blood Samples and Performing Injections

Some people dread the prick of blood glucose checks or insulin injections. These activities do not need to be excessively painful. Changing sites ("rotating sites") with each injection can help. Also, blood glucose levels can be checked by pricking the sides of the fingers if more comfortable and not just the pads, and less commonly, testing at other sites, such as the arms and legs, is possible. Be sure to ask your diabetes provider about other ways to minimize any pain.

When using needles to inject insulin, familiarity is key. Your provider can help you learn the proper technique and even provide very thin needles to ease this process. If you feel nervous about calculating the correct dose of insulin, ask for help. With proper training, injecting insulin can be relatively easy and very safe.

Social Support

Family and friends can be extremely valuable, but many people with diabetes find it helpful to reach beyond their usual social network to interact with others sharing similar health concerns (see "Social Support" on page 51). This is especially true for people who prefer not to share their diagnosis publicly.

Support groups organized specifically for people with diabetes offer an opportunity to share fears, celebrate triumphs, and work together on shared goals. These groups meet in person, online, or over the phone. Ask your provider for recommendations.

Planning for Problems

It's important to understand how and why emergencies happen, so don't be alarmed if your provider has a candid discussion with you about the potential dangers of diabetes. Even if you have no symptoms on most days, blood glucose levels can change quickly and lead to serious health problems. It's always important to follow your provider's instructions, take any prescribed medications as directed, and maintain the healthiest possible lifestyle.

WHAT DOES IT ALL MEAN?

- A diagnosis of diabetes requires ongoing education and changes in lifestyle, which can be overwhelming.
- Notify your provider of cultural practices and preferences in learning style, so he or she can develop the plan that works best for you.
- Ask for help with finger-stick blood glucose testing and injection techniques to reduce pain.

- Recognize that the emotional strain of diabetes is not uncommon and seek help from your diabetes care provider, therapists, or support groups.

Education in Diabetes Self-Management

Diabetes self-management education (DSME) refers to the ongoing process of acquiring the knowledge, skills, and abilities necessary for people with diabetes to care for their disease, with the goal of improving health for people with diabetes.

▶ WHAT YOU NEED TO KNOW

There's a lot to learn in the days and weeks following a diabetes diagnosis. People with diabetes and their caregivers must adjust to a new diet, new responsibilities, and a new daily routine. Some people must learn how to deliver insulin injections safely and effectively or monitor their blood glucose levels each day.

If you feel overwhelmed with these new tasks or would like to learn helpful strategies for common problems, ask your provider about attending a workshop or diabetes self-management educational classes. About half of all people with diabetes participate in these opportunities, and most people find them extremely helpful.

Educational Resources

- Ask your health care provider to refer you to a certified diabetes educator. These health care professionals have special training in diabetes education and can steer you through the ins and outs of diabetes care. This is especially helpful if you have other medical conditions or disabilities and need specialized advice. To find a clinical diabetes educator in your area, go to https://www.ncbde.org/find-a-cde/.
- Diabetes self-management training offers an interactive and fun approach to learning about how to care for diabetes at home. This program is typically taught by a nurse, dietitian, pharmacist, health care provider, or counselor who has special training in diabetes management. Contact your local diabetes clinic, pharmacy, or hospital to see if they offer this program. Participation is often reimbursed by insurance carriers or Medicare.
- Your provider may refer you to educational resources, such as handbooks or websites, that describe solutions to common issues encountered by people with diabetes.

The Lesson Plan

Most training courses cover the basic survival skills needed to manage diabetes at home. Here are a few common topics:

- ✓ How and when to take medications
- ✓ Common side effects of medications
- ✓ Insulin injections, storage, and needle disposal
- ✓ Using a glucose meter to record blood glucose levels at home
- ✓ Designing a healthy and tasty meal plan
- ✓ Recognizing and treating low blood glucose levels
- ✓ Setting personal goals for diet, exercise, and health
- ✓ Planning medical appointments
- ✓ When to call your provider

WHAT DOES IT ALL MEAN?

Learning diabetes management skills will provide you with the practical information you need to help treat your diabetes at home. You can discuss with your diabetes provider whether it would be best for you to meet one-on-one with a diabetes educator or attend a diabetes self-management course. DSME is critical for all people with diabetes to prevent or delay complications and may also be helpful for those with prediabetes to prevent progression to diabetes.

DIETARY THERAPY

Nutrition for Type 1 Diabetes

People with type 1 diabetes need to maintain a healthy, balanced diet that provides maximum nutrition. It will often focus on monitoring carbohydrate intake and sometimes, fat content. Proper nutrition is critical for effective type 1 diabetes management. Understanding how different foods, particularly carbohydrates, affect your blood glucose levels is important. Learning to develop balanced meal plans is a crucial part of the daily routine when living with type 1 diabetes.

▶ WHAT YOU NEED TO KNOW

Eating for Optimal Health in Type 1 Diabetes: Myths and Facts

MYTH: Meeting with a dietitian is only helpful when a person is first diagnosed with diabetes.

FACT: A dietitian can be helpful throughout a person's life. Newly diagnosed people with diabetes might work with a dietitian to learn the basics of carbohydrate counting and matching insulin doses to carbohydrate intake. Teenagers and young adults might learn how to boost their diet to enhance their growth and development. And people who have lived with the disease for many years might learn new and creative approaches to healthy eating or often benefit from a carbohydrate-counting refresher course.

MYTH: Low-carbohydrate diets are a necessity for all persons with type 1 diabetes.

FACT: Everyone eventually learns how to count the number of carbohydrates in their meals to determine the proper dose of insulin. The key then is not to necessarily restrict carbohydrates but to moderate carbohydrate intake and to inject the appropriate amount of insulin to cover the amount of carbs consumed.

MYTH: People with type 1 diabetes are limited to eating the same number of carbohydrates at each meal.

FACT: People who can count carbohydrates and calculate the correct dose of insulin can use a flexible insulin regimen based on the number of carbohydrates consumed. Using a personalized insulin-to-carbohydrate ratio allows you to calculate how much fast-acting, or nutritional, insulin to inject.

MYTH: People with type 1 diabetes are constantly at risk of dangerous high and low levels of blood glucose.

FACT: Many persons using insulin therapy are able to keep their blood glucose levels within a safe range. People can become experts in measuring the proper amount of insulin for the foods they eat, self-monitoring their blood glucose, and recognizing and preventing the earliest signs of low—or high—blood glucose before they occur. Diabetes education and working together with the health care team is critical.

WHAT DOES IT ALL MEAN?

Proper nutrition is important to the effective management of type 1 diabetes. From diagnosis, people with type 1 diabetes will be counseled on how to monitor and eventually count carbohydrates in their meal and adjust insulin doses accordingly. Meeting with a dietitian at any stage of the disease can be helpful.

After understanding core nutritional concepts, persons with type 1 diabetes can have flexible meal plans and enjoy a wide range of healthy and delicious foods.

Carbohydrate Counting

Carbohydrates are a major component of food that supply energy (*calories*) to the body. All foods contain one or more of the three major nutrients: carbohydrates, protein, and fat. Carbohydrates are present in different amounts in most foods, including fruits, vegetables, grains, beans, legumes, milk, and dairy products. They are also in foods containing added sugar (such as candy or soda). Types of carbohydrates include sugars, starches, and fiber. Counting grams of carbohydrate is often one of the first skills someone with type 1 diabetes will learn after diagnosis due to the effect of carbohydrates on blood glucose levels.

▶ WHAT YOU NEED TO KNOW

For both type 1 or type 2 diabetes, it's important to be aware of the number of carbohydrates in the foods you eat because they directly affect the rise in your blood glucose levels after meals. Carbohydrate counting is often discussed soon after diagnosis in persons with type 1 diabetes who are motivated and able to count the grams of carbohydrates in their meals. This requires working closely with the health care team, including a dietitian.

Foods such as candy, soda, fruit and fruit juice, milk, and yogurt contain sugar (*simple carbohydrates*) that is broken down easily and triggers a rapid rise in blood glucose levels. Complex carbohydrates, such as whole grains or starchy vegetables, take longer to break down, allowing for a slow, steady rise in blood glucose levels after meals. Dietary fiber includes the parts of plant foods that your body can't digest or absorb but that may have other benefits, such as lowering blood cholesterol or glucose, maintaining bowel health, and making you feel full.

Understanding the Nutrition Facts

Carbohydrate counting begins with the food package label. When you examine a label, start by looking at the number of servings per package. Remember that some packages may contain more than one serving, even if it looks to be an individual serving (such as a bag of chips or a bottle of soda). Second, look for the grams of total carbohydrates. Every 15 grams of carbohydrates is considered 1 *carb serving*, regardless of where the carbohydrate comes from (whether it's a piece of bread or a box of raisins). A carbohydrate serving is different from the *serving size* listed on the label. A product's serving size simply refers to the amount normally eaten by the average individual. You may be eating more than the suggested serving size, which means that you will have to calculate the total number of grams that are actually in your meal.

For example, a box of cereal states that one serving of the cereal is 1 cup. In that 1 cup, there are 30 grams of carbohydrate. If you plan to eat 1½ cups, you will need to figure out how many grams of carbohydrate are in ½ cup. Take the grams (30) and divide by 2. This will give you the amount of carbohydrate in ½ cup (15 grams). Take this amount and add it to the amount of carbohydrate in 1 cup: 30 + 15 = 45 grams of carbohydrate in 1½ cups of the cereal.

To learn more about how to use nutrition facts labels to count your carbohydrates, it may be helpful to meet with a registered dietitian to practice.

Recognizing Single Servings

As you practice and become a more skilled carb counter, you'll learn to recognize single (15 gram) carbohydrate servings. Here are a few examples of 15-gram carbohydrates (or 1 carb serving):

Starches and Grains
- one-third of a medium bagel
- one slice of sandwich bread
- ¾ cup cold unsweetened cereal
- ⅓ cup pasta or rice

Fruits
- one-half of a medium banana
- one small apple
- 2 tbsp dried fruit
- 17 grapes
- 1 cup melon
- ¾ cup berries

Sweets
- two small cookies
- five vanilla wafers
- ½ cup sugar-free pudding

Combination Foods
- ½ cup casserole

- one-half of a sandwich
- one small taco

Dairy
- 1 cup milk
- small cup plain yogurt

WHAT DOES IT ALL MEAN?

Carbohydrate counting is a skill that persons with type 1 diabetes (and some people with type 2 diabetes using mealtime insulin) need to learn while working closely with their dietitian. Awareness of the carbohydrate content of meals is important for persons with all types of diabetes since carbohydrate intake can greatly affect blood glucose levels. By learning to count carbohydrates in meals, people with diabetes can have improved and more predictable blood glucose levels.

Nutrition for Type 2 Diabetes

A healthy diet is essential for managing type 2 diabetes for many reasons. The foods consumed can have a significant impact on blood glucose levels. In addition, people with type 2 diabetes often need to lose weight to help improve the body's response to insulin and to reduce the risks of complications such as heart disease. A diet low in calories, consistent in carbohydrates (or moderate in carbohydrates), and a regular exercise routine are vital to managing type 2 diabetes. A healthy diet usually consists of eating fewer calories and processed foods and controlling portions of the daily intake from all the food groups, with an emphasis on eating more nonstarchy vegetables.

▶ WHAT YOU NEED TO KNOW

Eating for Optimal Health in Type 2 Diabetes: Myths and Facts

MYTH: Weight loss can reduce the need for type 2 diabetes treatment but only if there is a dramatic change.

FACT: Many people who are overweight or obese develop type 2 diabetes. Often, people find that losing even a modest amount of weight (5% to 7%) reduces the doses and number of diabetes medications required and in rare cases can result in diabetes being well managed without the need for medication altogether.

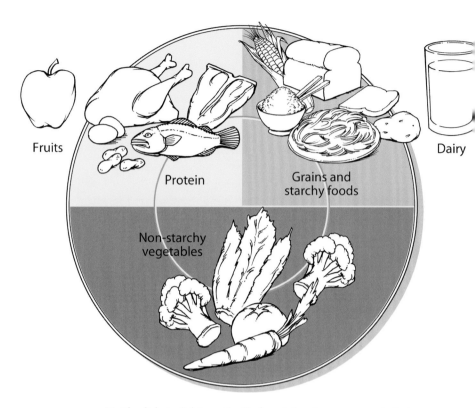

Fruits

Protein

Grains and
starchy foods

Dairy

Non-starchy
vegetables

5.1 The diabetes "plate method" of meal planning recommends that half the meal consist of nonstarchy vegetables, a quarter consist of protein, and a quarter consist of grains or starchy foods. A serving of fruit or dairy can also be added. © 2018, Johns Hopkins University, Art as Applied to Medicine

MYTH: Meeting with a dietitian is only helpful when a person is first diagnosed with diabetes.

FACT: Newly diagnosed people often work with a dietitian to learn the basics of carbohydrate awareness and making healthy food choices. However, a dietitian can be helpful at any stage of the disease to help manage blood glucose levels and complications related to diabetes (such as diabetic kidney disease), to assist in weight loss, and to help the person with diabetes manage blood sugars by eating consistent amounts of carbohydrate throughout the day.

MYTH: Low-carbohydrate diets are a must for all persons with type 2 diabetes.

FACT: Persons with type 2 diabetes should be aware of the carbohydrates in their diet and not overindulge or restrict excessively. Beyond that, more research is needed about whether it's beneficial to limit specific types of foods or aim for certain proportions of the three macronutrients (that is, fats, proteins, and carbohydrates) in each meal. One thing the studies do agree on, however, is that a strategy of reducing calories is important for weight loss success. The diabetes plate method is often recommended for people with all types of diabetes (figure 5.1). This method estimates that if a meal is placed on a 9-inch round plate, one-half of the plate should be filled with nonstarchy vegetables, one-fourth of the plate should be protein, and one-fourth of the plate should be grains and starchy foods. An additional serving of fruit or dairy may also be included. This method of eating can be helpful because as long as you watch portion sizes, this meal plan provides consistent amounts of carbohydrate. Talk to your dietitian about what method best suits your needs.

MYTH: When reading food package labels, persons with diabetes should focus on the number of carbohydrates. The nutritional content can be disregarded.

FACT: While monitoring carbohydrate intake is clearly important, dietitians may also recommend limiting calories, sodium, and saturated fats. Avoid trans fats whenever possible. People with diabetes are encouraged to eat a diet rich in fiber and choose complex carbohydrates—whole-grain bread and vegetables— over the simple sugars found in table sugar, sugar-sweetened beverages, and candy.

WHAT DOES IT ALL MEAN?

- Everyone has individual needs. Work with your provider, registered dietitian, or diabetes educator to develop a meal plan that works for you.
- Take time to plan your meals according to the diabetes plate method and pay attention to the number of calories, the healthy fats, the grams of fiber, and the carbohydrate content.
- You can still eat out at restaurants, but be aware of the nutritional content of your meals; many restaurants provide this information online, at the point of service, or upon request.

Sugar Substitutes and Artificial Sweeteners

Sugar substitutes refer to any sweetener that is used in foods instead of regular table sugar (sucrose). There are two main types of sweeteners: natural and artificial. Natural (or *nutritive*) sweeteners provide energy in the form of carbohydrates. Artificial (or *nonnutritive*) sweeteners do not contain carbohydrates and have low to no calories. While people with diabetes do not necessarily need to use sugar substitutes or artificial sweeteners, food or drinks that contain them may be an option to help curb cravings for sweets.

▶ WHAT YOU NEED TO KNOW

Natural sweeteners include sugars such as glucose, sucrose, or fructose that are found naturally in fruits, vegetables, and other plants. These include honey, agave nectar, or maple syrup. Artificial sweeteners are man-made and are not usually derived from plants or other foods. Artificial sweeteners are many times sweeter than regular sugar and are widely used in processed and sugar-free foods, including baked goods, soft drinks, candy, and many other foods and beverages.

When you sweeten your morning coffee, what do you reach for? If you're like most people, you're probably loyal to a certain color—perhaps you prefer blue packets of sweetener, or maybe pink. But have you given thought to what those colors mean? Table 5.1 contains a list of some common sweeteners you might encounter.

WHAT DOES IT ALL MEAN?

- Never assume that a food labeled "sugar-free," "no sugar added," or "low calorie" doesn't contain carbohydrates.
- Foods with these labels may still contain natural sweeteners that have calories called *sugar alcohols*, such as sorbitol, xylitol, mannitol, erythritol, glycerol, or hydrogenated starch hydrolysates. Be careful when consuming foods containing sugar alcohols, as eating too much of them may cause digestive discomfort such as gas, bloating, abdominal cramping, and diarrhea.
- Always count the number of carbohydrates on the nutrition label rather than assuming a food can be eaten freely.
- Foods and drinks advertised as "diet," "low-calorie," and "sugar-free" can help with weight loss, as long as you don't overeat them.
- Artificial sweeteners don't usually noticeably raise blood glucose levels and may be a good alternative for persons with diabetes. However, some research suggests that these sweeteners may be related to weight gain for reasons that are unclear.

Table 5.1. Common artificial sweeteners

NAME	COLOR	SWEETENER	SWEETNESS INDEX
Equal, NutraSweet	Blue packets	Contains the artificial sweetener *aspartame*	About 200 times sweeter than sugar
Splenda	Yellow packets	Contains the artificial sweetener *sucralose*	About 600 times sweeter than sugar
Sweet 'N Low (also Necta Sweet)	Pink packets	Contains the artificial sweetener *saccharin*	About 200–700 times sweeter than sugar
Truvia, PureVia, SweetLeaf	Green-and-white packets	Contains the natural sweetener *stevia*, extracted from the stevia leaf	About 200–400 times sweeter than sugar
Sweet One, Sunett	Multicolored packets	Contains the artificial sweetener *acesulfame potassium*	About 200 times sweeter than sugar
Newtame	White packets	Contains the artificial sweetener *neotame*	About 7,000–13,000 times sweeter than sugar

Popular Diets and Weight Loss Programs

Many American adults struggle with weight loss. For people with diabetes, this is a worthy battle: small-to-moderate amounts of weight loss—just 5% to 7%—can dramatically improve blood glucose control and reduce your need for diabetes medications.

Many people tackle the weight-loss journey on their own, setting out to cut calories, choose healthy foods, and set aside time for exercise. However, others prefer more structured weight-loss programs to help them lose weight.

► WHAT YOU NEED TO KNOW

Joining a structured weight-loss program can help you shed your body weight. There are many programs to choose from. Some are commercial, meaning you pay to join a group of other dieters who have a leader, or coach. Others are free, meaning you can read about them and start anytime without paying a fee.

Some diets focus on eliminating or restricting a certain component of food, like carbs or fat, while others simply focus on counting calories.

There is no single best diet for people with diabetes. Rather than opting for the most popular option, choose a diet that easily matches your schedule, respects your cultural and behavioral preferences, and honors your personal taste.

Free (Noncommercial) Diet Plans
Plans That Limit Fat

- The *Dietary Approaches to Stop Hypertension (DASH)* diet cuts back on foods that are high in saturated fat and limits red meat, salt, sweets, and sugary drinks. It encourages dieters to eat fruits, vegetables, whole-grain foods, fish, poultry, nuts, and low-fat dairy products. This diet has been shown to lower blood pressure.

- The *Dean Ornish Diet* allows dieters to eat carbohydrates and consume very little fat. This diet may help reverse the damage to the arteries in people with coronary atherosclerosis. Those with diabetes may have a difficult time with this diet, as carbohydrates raise blood glucose.

- The *Pritikin Weight Loss Breakthrough* encourages dieters to consume less than 10% of their daily calories from fat, which is thought to improve cholesterol levels.

- The *Therapeutic Lifestyle Changes (TLC)* diet focuses on reducing the amount of saturated fats in the diet (such as fatty meats, whole-fat dairy, and fried foods), as well as trans fats, to lower cholesterol levels.

Plans That Limit Carbohydrates

- The *Atkins* and *South Beach Diets* restrict carbohydrates dramatically at first and then gradually reintroduce carbohydrates into the meal plan. Both diets lead to weight loss, but few studies have looked at the long-term success of the South Beach Diet. People who choose the Atkins Diet generally see the same amount of improvement in their blood glucose levels as they might see by enrolling in dietary counseling.

- The *Zone Diet* encourages dieters to reduce overall calories and design meal plans that are made up of 30% proteins, 30% fats, and 40% carbohydrates. Dieters generally do lose weight, but it's unclear whether the Zone Diet has long-term benefits for blood glucose control.
- The glycemic index (GI) can be incorporated into meal plans and is based on how certain foods affect your blood glucose levels. Many other diets incorporate this system.
  - Generally, foods with a *high* GI (such as mashed potatoes) contain a lot of carbohydrates and cause blood glucose levels to "spike," or rise quickly. Foods with a *low* GI (such as kidney beans) have few carbohydrates and have a milder effect on blood glucose levels.
  - Some people lose weight faster—and have healthier blood glucose levels—when they stick to a low GI diet.

Other Diet Plans
- The *Mediterranean Diet* emphasizes eating primarily plant-based foods, such as fruits and vegetables, whole grains, and legumes and nuts, and replacing butter with healthier fats, such as olive oil. The diet also recommends limiting red meat to no more than a few times a month and eating fish at least twice a week. Studies have shown that the Mediterranean Diet may reduce the risk of heart disease.
- The *American Diabetes Association (ADA)* recommends an individualized medical nutrition strategy, preferably provided by a registered dietitian. This often includes limiting calories and portion control. Carbohydrate intake from whole grains, vegetables, fruit, legumes, and dairy products is emphasized, with no ideal dietary distribution of carbohydrates, fats, and proteins. This diet limits salt and saturated fats and encourages the intake of fiber. This not only promotes healthy blood glucose levels but may also reduce your risk of heart disease by improving your blood pressure. A variety of eating patterns may be helpful for people with diabetes, including the Mediterranean Diet, DASH Diet, or plant-based diets.

Commercial (Paid) Diet Plans
Weight Watchers
- Dieters track and limit calories daily using a points system.
- Dieters prepare their own meals and snacks. No foods are restricted, but less-healthy options use up more points out of the daily allowance.
- The plan recommends eating twice as many carbohydrates and fats as proteins.

- This program describes the diet as easy to follow. This diet has shown that members can achieve effective weight loss in the first few months. Studies have shown that dieters lose up to 3% more weight than nondieters after 1 year.
- No studies have looked at A1C levels in people with diabetes who follow the Weight Watchers program.

Jenny Craig
- Dieters replace traditional meals with low-calorie bars, drinks, or meals. Most meals and snacks are provided by the company.
- The program states that users lose an average of 1 to 2 pounds per week. Studies have shown that dieters lost about 5% more weight than nondieters after 1 year.
- After 6 months, A1C levels dropped a bit more in people who followed the Jenny Craig diet compared with those who only received dietary counseling in research studies.

Nutrisystem
- Dieters replace traditional meals with low-calorie bars, drinks, or meals and eat smaller balanced meals six times a day. Most meals and snacks are provided by the company.
- The program states that dieters can expect to lose 1 to 2 pounds per week. Studies have shown that after 3 to 6 months, dieters lost up to 5% more weight than nondieters.
- After 6 months, A1C levels dropped a bit more in people who used Nutrisystem compared with those who only received dietary counseling in research studies.

WHAT DOES IT ALL MEAN?
- Weight loss can have a dramatic positive effect on treating diabetes.
- Some people can lose weight by simply eating less and increasing their physical activity. Others prefer more structured diet plans.
- Meeting with a dietitian can be useful in deciding which meal plan to choose.
- Using a food log or mobile application to track dietary intake can be helpful for many people with diabetes to lose weight.
- Many commercial diet plans exist. However, these are paid weight-loss programs. Talk to your health care provider to see if these programs or meal replacements might be a good fit for you.

EXERCISE

Physical Activity and Exercise

Physical activity is a general term that refers to any movement that increases the use of energy by the body. Exercise is a specific form of physical activity that is more planned and structured and intended to improve physical fitness. Both physical activity and exercise are critical components of an effective diabetes management plan.

▶ WHAT YOU NEED TO KNOW

Did you know that regular exercise can have many significant health benefits for persons with diabetes? Many people think they need to carve out a major portion of their daily schedule to make room for a vigorous, time-intensive exercise regimen. But the reality is that a simple combination of aerobic activity and weight training can improve how you feel, inside and out. Regular exercise makes a difference by

- improving blood glucose levels, blood pressure, and cholesterol;
- improving mood and potentially reducing the chance of depression;
- trimming the waistline and reducing body fat;
- lowering the risk of heart disease;
- possibly reducing the need or doses for diabetes medications; and
- preventing or delaying type 2 diabetes development in persons with prediabetes.

The first rule of the game is to set achievable goals. Begin by exercising a few days a week. Once you notice the effects of physical activity on your health and body shape, you'll likely be motivated to increase the frequency and intensity of your exercise regimen. Until then, don't sweat it! Here are some other helpful tips.

Types of Exercise

- Persons with diabetes benefit most from a combination of aerobic exercise and resistance training (figure 5.2).
- Aerobic activity raises the heart rate through upbeat, rhythmic movement. Examples include walking, cycling, jogging, and swimming.
- Resistance (strength) training strengthens the muscles. Examples include activities such as Pilates; yoga; or exercises using free weights, weight machines, body weight, or elastic resistance bands.
- For persons with type 1 or type 2 diabetes, 150 minutes or more of aerobic

exercise and two to three sessions of resistance exercise per week is generally recommended.

- Flexibility and balance training may be particularly important for older adults with diabetes to improve the range of motion around joints and prevent falls.
- Avoid going more than 2 days in a row without exercise.
- If 30-minute workouts are too intense or you have trouble making time for them, try scattering three 10-minute sessions throughout the day. You might find it much easier to follow through with your fitness goals.
- In addition to exercise, breaking up the amount of time spent sitting during the day by briefly standing, walking, or performing other light activities every 30 minutes can have health benefits, especially in persons with type 2 diabetes.

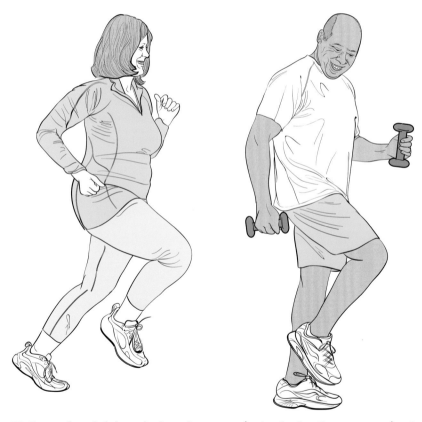

5.2 For people with diabetes, both aerobic exercise (such as brisk walking or jogging) and resistance exercise (such as weight lifting) are important for optimal health and diabetes management. © 2018, Johns Hopkins University, Art as Applied to Medicine

- Invite a friend, join a class, or work with a personal trainer. People who have strong social support are more likely than others to stick to their routines.
- Find a physical activity you *enjoy*! Remember—exercise only works if you do it. If the exercise you choose is fun, you're not only more likely to do it but to have fun doing it.

Adjustments to Diabetes Management
- Exercise lowers blood glucose. If you have insulin-treated diabetes, ask your provider if your dose of insulin should be decreased on the days that you exercise.
- Check your blood glucose levels before and after exercise to become familiar with your body's responses to various types of activity. For example, your blood glucose might respond differently to lifting weights than it would to a pickup basketball game. Changes in blood glucose levels (high or low) can sometimes last several hours after exercise.
- Working out causes your body to burn blood glucose. For that reason, persons with diabetes may need to eat a small snack before and after exercise. Always keep a snack on hand in case your blood glucose drops too low.

Special Precautions
- Always check with your health care provider before starting a new exercise routine to be safe.
- Stay hydrated. Drink plenty of fluids before, during, and after exercise.
- Check your feet daily for blisters or other signs of injury. Discuss nonhealing injuries with your health care provider as soon as you notice them.
- Watch for symptoms of heart disease, which may include lightheadedness; shortness of breath; and chest pressure, pain, or tightness. Stop exercise immediately and alert your health care provider.
- Stop exercising if you feel lightheaded or dizzy or have other signs of low blood pressure.
- Keep treatment for low blood glucose levels with you when you exercise. Examples include glucose tablets, juice boxes, or hard candy.
- Wear diabetes identification—especially if you are exercising alone.

WHAT DOES IT ALL MEAN?

A combination of aerobic exercise and weight training can improve blood glucose levels and offer several other health benefits, including mood-boosting effects, improvement in blood glucose levels, and possibly weight loss. Workout routines do not need to be elaborate or time intensive; even three 10-minute intervals spread throughout the day can start you off on the right foot. People who have not exercised regularly should talk to their health care provider before starting an exercise program. Those who are at especially high risk for cardiovascular complications or who have a previous history of heart disease or stroke might need a stress test before beginning an exercise regimen.

Chapter 6

OBESITY AND DIABETES

Managing Obesity

Obesity is a disease associated with having too much body fat. People are generally considered obese when their body mass index (BMI), a measurement obtained by dividing their weight (in kilograms) by the square of their height (in meters), is 30 kg/m² or over. The range of 25 to 29.9 kg/m² is defined as overweight. However, in Asians a BMI of 27.5 kg/m² or above is considered obese, and 23 to 27.4 kg/m² is considered overweight.

▶ WHAT YOU NEED TO KNOW

Nearly two-thirds of all U.S. adults are overweight or obese. Table 6.1 provides a reference chart to calculate body mass index based on height and weight and indicates the overweight and obese ranges for the general population (for Asians these cutoffs are lower). Obesity is also increasing in other parts of the world. Obesity management can delay the progression from prediabetes to diabetes and is especially beneficial in the treatment of type 2 diabetes. Sustained weight loss can improve blood glucose, triglycerides, blood pressure, and abnormal cholesterol levels (*dyslipidemia*) and potentially reduce the need for medications in persons with type 2 diabetes.

Exercise and a Healthy Diet
   Regardless of which diet makes the most headlines, the key to losing weight will always be a reduced-calorie diet and regular physical activity (see "Physical Activity and Exercise" on page 95 and "Nutrition for Type 2 Diabetes" on page 87). Dietitians can help design an individualized meal plan and give referrals to a comprehensive weight management program.

Table 6.1. Calculation of body mass index by height and weight (kg/m^2)

	100 LBS	110 LBS	120 LBS	130 LBS	140 LBS	150 LBS	160 LBS	170 LB
4'8"	22	25	26	29	31	34	36	38
4'9"	22	24	26	28	30	33	35	37
4'10"	21	23	25	27	29	31	34	36
4'11"	20	22	24	26	28	30	32	34
5'0"	20	22	23	25	27	29	31	33
5'1"	19	21	23	25	26	28	30	32
5'2"	18	20	22	24	26	27	29	31
5'3"	18	20	21	23	25	27	28	30
5'4"		19	21	22	24	26	28	29
5'5"		18	20	22	23	25	27	28
5'6"		18	19	21	23	24	26	27
5'7"			19	20	22	24	25	27
5'8"			18	20	22	23	24	26
5'9"			18	19	21	22	24	25
5'10"			17	19	20	22	23	24
5'11"			17	18	20	21	22	24
6'0"			16	18	19	20	22	23
6'1"			16	17	19	20	21	22
	45 KG	50 KG	54 KG	59 KG	63 KG	68 KG	73 KG	77 KG

Note: kg/m^2 = kilograms per square meter.

LBS	190 LBS	200 LBS	210 LBS	220 LBS	230 LBS	240 LBS	250 LBS	
40	43	45	47	49	52	54	56	146 cm
39	41	43	45	48	50	52	54	147 cm
38	40	42	44	46	48	50	52	149 cm
36	38	40	42	44	46	49	51	150 cm
35	37	39	41	43	45	47	49	152 cm
34	36	38	40	42	44	45	47	155 cm
33	35	37	38	40	42	44	46	157 cm
32	34	35	37	39	41	43	44	160 cm
31	33	34	36	38	40	41	43	163 cm
30	33	33	35	37	38	40	42	165 cm
29	31	32	34	36	37	39	40	167 cm
28	30	31	33	35	36	38	39	170 cm
27	29	30	32	34	35	37	38	173 cm
27	28	30	31	33	34	35	37	175 cm
26	27	29	30	32	33	35	36	178 cm
25	27	28	29	31	32	34	35	180 cm
24	26	27	28	30	31	33	34	183 cm
24	25	26	28	29	30	32	33	185 cm
KG	86 KG	91 KG	95 KG	100 KG	104 KG	109 KG	113 KG	

eral BMI cutoffs (shown above): <25 kg/m^2 = healthy weight (white),
29.9 kg/m^2 = overweight (medium blue), ≥30 kg/m^2 = obese (dark blue)

cutoffs for Asians: <23 kg/m^2 = healthy weight, 23–27.4 kg/m^2 = overweight,
.5 kg/m^2 = obese

Medications for Weight Loss

In addition to diet and physical activity, prescription weight-loss drugs can offer modest weight loss (usually 5% to 10% of total body weight) in persons with diabetes who are obese and in some persons who are overweight. However, most people will eventually gain the weight back once they stop taking the drug if they don't continue to follow a healthy lifestyle. Some examples of weight-loss drugs for long-term use (more than a few weeks) include the following:

- *Orlistat* (brand names Alli or Xenical) works by preventing the body from absorbing fats. Side effects may include oily diarrhea, gas, and stomach cramping.
- *Phentermine/topiramate ER* (brand name Qsymia) works in the brain to reduce appetite. Side effects may include dizziness, drowsiness, difficulty sleeping, constipation, headache, dryness in the mouth, and numbness or tingling in the hands or feet. This medication can cause birth defects and should not be used during pregnancy.
- *Lorcaserin* (brand name Belviq) acts on the brain to reduce appetite, leading to weight loss. Side effects may include headaches, low blood glucose, and fatigue.
- *Naltrexone/buproprion* (brand name Contrave) is a medication that also works in the brain to affect the appetite and produce weight loss. Side effects may include nausea, constipation, headache, and vomiting.
- *Liraglutide* (brand name Saxenda) is a GLP-1 receptor agonist that is also approved for the treatment of diabetes. At higher doses, it is approved as a stand-alone drug for weight loss in people with or without diabetes. The higher the liraglutide dose, the higher the expected weight loss. Side effects may include low blood glucose, nausea, vomiting, diarrhea, constipation, and headache.

Weight-Loss Surgery

After trying medical management, people who are very obese may opt for surgery to lose weight (see "Bariatric Surgery" on page 103). These operations can lead to dramatic weight loss and improvements in blood glucose, blood pressure, and cholesterol levels in persons with type 2 diabetes who are considered good candidates for this surgery. In some cases, remission of diabetes is also possible. However, weight-loss surgery carries potential complications, such as lifelong vitamin and mineral deficiencies, and sustained weight loss after bariatric surgery can be a challenge. To achieve the best outcomes, people undergoing bariatric surgery must commit to a permanent healthy lifestyle.

Many people with type 2 diabetes struggle with their body weight. With regular physical exercise and a healthy portion-controlled diet, weight loss will occur, but it may not always be sufficient or long lasting. Losing just 5% to 7% of your total body weight can dramatically lower your risk of developing type 2 diabetes or reduce the amount of medications you need if you already have diabetes. Keeping the weight off is just as important as losing the weight in the first place, so commit to a healthy lifestyle for the long run. If you've been unsuccessful in losing weight with lifestyle management or medications, consider talking to your medical team about surgical options.

Bariatric Surgery

Bariatric (or metabolic) surgery can help some people with type 2 diabetes and obesity lose weight and improve their diabetes by making anatomical changes to the digestive system. Some types of bariatric surgery make the stomach smaller, leading to the sensation of feeling full sooner. Other bariatric surgeries shorten the small intestine—the part of the body that absorbs calories and nutrients from foods and beverages.

▶ WHAT YOU NEED TO KNOW

When diet, exercise, or weight-loss medications aren't effective for losing weight, some people turn to weight-loss surgery, also known as bariatric surgery. These procedures can dramatically improve blood glucose levels in some people with type 2 diabetes who have obesity and most often lead to a reduced need for medications or, in some cases, complete remission.

Is Weight-Loss Surgery Right for You?

A person's BMI is calculated first to determine if weight-loss surgery is appropriate. BMI is a way of looking at both height and weight and classifying people as underweight, healthy, or overweight (Table 6.1).

Weight-loss surgery is generally recommended for

- people with diabetes who are extremely obese (usually a BMI of 40 kg/m^2 or greater; in Asians, a BMI of 37.5 kg/m^2 or greater)

or

- persons who are obese (usually a BMI of 35 kg/m^2 or greater; in Asians, a BMI of 32.5 kg/m^2 or greater) with poorly managed diabetes despite medical management.

Persons with diabetes who are obese (usually a BMI of 30 kg/m² or greater; in Asians, a BMI of 27.5 kg/m² or greater) should talk to their health care provider about whether they may also be considered surgical candidates.

Common Types of Weight-Loss Surgery

Laparoscopic adjustable gastric band An adjustable band is slipped around part of the stomach. The band can be made looser or tighter after the surgery. As a result, the stomach is smaller and holds less food, leading to weight loss.

Laparoscopic sleeve gastrectomy The surgeon removes a large part of the stomach, making it smaller. It therefore can hold less food after the surgery, leading to weight loss.

Roux-en-Y gastric bypass This surgery takes a two-step approach to weight loss. First, it makes the stomach smaller. Second, it reduces the amount of food the body can digest by shortening the small intestine, leading to weight loss.

What Can People Expect after Surgery?

Most people will notice dramatic improvements in blood glucose levels, even before any weight loss occurs. Improvements in blood pressure and cholesterol levels can also occur. People who take insulin or pills for diabetes often find they require much lower doses or sometimes can stop their medications. Blood glucose levels often become easier to manage over time. Some studies suggest that bariatric surgery may also reduce complications from diabetes and help prevent heart disease and death.

However, bariatric surgery has potential drawbacks, including complications related to the surgical procedure itself. Bariatric surgery is also costly and may have side effects, including long-term nutritional deficiencies in important vitamins and minerals (such as vitamin D) that require lifelong supplementation. *Dumping syndrome*, or rapid gastric emptying after surgery, may lead to symptoms of nausea, vomiting, abdominal pain and cramping, and diarrhea—particularly after eating foods rich in simple sugars or carbohydrates. Hypoglycemia after meals (see "Hypoglycemia after Meals" on page 41) may also occur after Roux-en-Y gastric bypass surgery.

WHAT DOES IT ALL MEAN?

The benefits of weight-loss surgery are exciting, and it may be a helpful option in adults with obesity who struggle with managing their type 2 diabetes despite taking their medications and making lifestyle changes. People with diabetes considering bariatric surgery should, in consultation with their health care team, carefully weigh its potential short- and long-term complications and the need for ongoing monitoring before making a final decision.

Chapter 7

DIABETES COMPLICATIONS AND OTHER CONDITIONS COMMON IN DIABETES

THE BRAIN

Stroke

Cerebrovascular diseases refer to medical conditions, such as stroke, that result in a disruption of blood flow to the brain. A stroke is a serious medical condition in which a blood vessel is blocked—most commonly by a blood clot—causing a lack of blood flow, and therefore oxygen, to the brain (ischemic stroke). A stroke can also result when a blood vessel bursts, and bleeding damages the surrounding brain tissue (hemorrhagic stroke). In general, ischemic strokes are more common than hemorrhagic strokes. In addition, ischemic strokes are more common in people with diabetes than in people without diabetes.

▶ WHAT YOU NEED TO KNOW

People with type 2 diabetes are more than two times likely than others to have an ischemic stroke. That's not surprising when you consider that many of the risk factors for stroke and diabetes overlap, including hypertension, high cholesterol, and obesity (figure 7.2).

What Are the Warning Signs of a Stroke?

The symptoms of a stroke can come on suddenly, without warning. If you notice any of the following symptoms, particularly in a person with diabetes, call for emergency medical assistance:

- Numbness or weakness, often on one side of the body
- Trouble speaking

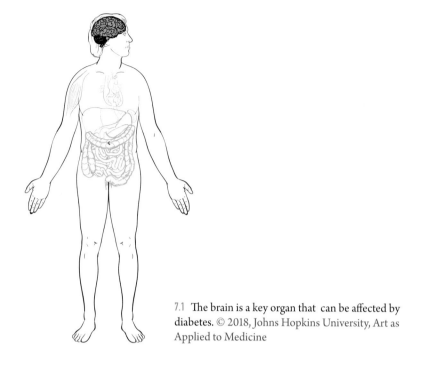

7.1 The brain is a key organ that can be affected by diabetes. © 2018, Johns Hopkins University, Art as Applied to Medicine

- Trouble understanding speech
- Dizziness
- Problems walking
- Visual disturbances
- Nausea, possibly with vomiting
- Headache

Some of these symptoms can also occur with hypoglycemia, so it is important to ensure that blood glucose levels are not low when you are having these symptoms.

What Tests Are Done to Confirm a Stroke?

It is important to go to the emergency room immediately if a stroke is suspected to identify and treat it as quickly as possible. Early treatment can limit the extent of damage to the brain. When health care providers suspect that someone has had a stroke, a CT scan or an MRI is performed immediately to help determine if the stroke was hemorrhagic or ischemic. In a subset of people who present with an ischemic stroke within 3 hours, and sometimes up to 4.5 hours, treatment with intravenous recombinant tissue plasminogen activator (tPA) may dramatically reduce the amount of brain damage and improve recovery. In

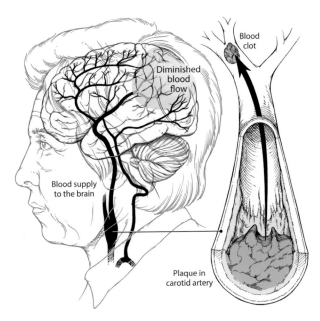

7.2 In an ischemic stroke, blood supply to a part of the brain is blocked due to a clot in the blood vessels. © 2018, Johns Hopkins University, Art as Applied to Medicine

some cases, a clot may be seen on an *angiogram* of the brain and can be removed directly from the blocked blood vessel in the brain during a procedure called a *thrombectomy*. However, this can usually only be done within the first 6 hours after symptom onset and only after receiving tPA. Since treatments to dissolve dangerous clots in the blood vessels can only be performed within the first few hours, it is vital to go to the emergency room as soon as a stroke is suspected. Even when a person is not a candidate for these immediate treatments, further testing must be performed to determine the cause of the stroke and to start other treatments that can prevent another stroke. In some cases, blood tests may reveal that a person has an entirely different condition, often treatable, that mimics the symptoms of stroke.

How Can I Prevent a Stroke?

Fortunately, there are several healthy changes that you can make to lower your risk of a stroke:

- Better manage your blood glucose levels. Studies have shown that stroke may occur less often in people with better blood glucose management.
- Lower your blood pressure. Treating high blood pressure can lower your risk of stroke dramatically.

Diabetes Complications and Other Conditions

- Treat high cholesterol. Ask your health care provider for help lowering your bad cholesterol and raising your good cholesterol. If healthy lifestyle changes don't work, medications are available. However, most people with diabetes aged 40 years and older should already be on a statin medication to prevent strokes from occurring in the first place (see "Statins" on page 277).
- Stop smoking. People who smoke have a dramatically higher risk of stroke (and heart disease). Ask your health care provider for help to stop smoking.
- Aspirin therapy. Many people with diabetes may benefit from a low-dose aspirin. Ask your health care provider if aspirin therapy is right for you.
- Adopt a healthy lifestyle. Exercising regularly and following a healthy eating plan are important. If you are overweight or obese, weight loss can also be beneficial.

WHAT DOES IT ALL MEAN?

Strokes are a serious medical condition that occur more often in people with diabetes. Long-term effects after a stroke can include impaired vision or speech, severe weakness or paralysis on one side of the body, swallowing difficulties, memory loss, depression, and mood swings. Strokes can lead to significant disability in the day-to-day life of people with diabetes. Many steps can be taken to prevent you from having a stroke or to reverse the damage from having a stroke. Whenever a stroke is suspected, immediate medical attention is critical.

Dementia and Neurodegenerative Diseases

Neurodegenerative diseases are incurable and debilitating medical conditions in which nerve cells gradually deteriorate or die. Illnesses that cause progressive memory loss along with other cognitive and personality changes are referred to as *dementia*. There are several types of dementia. The most common of these is Alzheimer disease, which accounts for half of all cases. Another common type is vascular dementia. People with diabetes are at higher risk of developing both types of dementia.

▶ WHAT YOU NEED TO KNOW

In today's world, it is common for older people to develop dementia, a gradual cognitive (or mental) decline marked by personality changes and memory loss. Though dementia is a concern for any older adult, it can be especially worrisome for people with diabetes. Older people with diabetes face about a two-fold higher risk of dementia.

What Causes Cognitive Decline?

A number of factors are known to contribute to cognitive decline in people with diabetes. This risk is higher in people who have had a previous stroke or have underlying heart disease. People with type 2 diabetes tend to be overweight or obese or have other conditions such as high blood pressure or high cholesterol, which puts them at increased risk for vascular dementia, a type of dementia that results from multiple small strokes.

While persistently higher blood glucose levels over time may contribute to cognitive decline, the impact of low blood glucose levels (hypoglycemia) is not as clear. Though people with type 1 diabetes who experience repeated episodes of low blood glucose are prone to confusion and difficulty concentrating, they were not any more likely to have long-term cognitive decline in the Diabetes Complications and Control Trial (see "Landmark Studies in Diabetes Care" on page 6). Also, very intensive treatments to lower blood glucose levels were not necessarily related to changes in cognitive function among people with type 2 diabetes in the ACCORD study (see "Landmark Studies in Diabetes Care" on page 6).

How Do Health Care Providers Diagnose Dementia?

To determine if a person has dementia, the health care provider will do a complete exam, including blood tests and brain imaging, to rule out other illnesses. The provider might also ask the patient and a family member or caretaker many questions to determine how well the patient can speak, remember basic information, recognize objects and people, move around, and coordinate actions. Sometimes a full series of cognitive or mental tests are performed, which may need to be repeated at intervals to determine if cognition is progressively declining.

Based on the results of these tests, the provider may diagnose the patient with dementia.

How Is Dementia Treated?

Unfortunately, scientists are still searching for effective treatments for dementia. Some drugs, such as cholinesterase inhibitors (donepezil, rivastigmine, or galantamine, for example) have been shown to slow the progression of Alzheimer disease somewhat. The side effects of these drugs can include nausea, vomiting, and diarrhea and may not be tolerable for all people. However, there is no known cure for dementia.

Dementia is a common problem among older adults. People with diabetes are at higher risk. Dementia can progress over many years, and there is currently no cure, but a few medications are available to help with symptoms. If you are having problems with memory, confusion, or concentration, talk to your health care provider to see if you need further testing.

Depression

Depression (*major depressive disorder* or *clinical depression*) is a common and serious mood disorder related to a persistent feeling of sadness and a loss of interest in one's usual activities. It can affect how a person feels, thinks, and behaves and can lead to other emotional and physical problems. Difficulty with normal day-to-day activities, such as sleeping, eating, or working, and a feeling that life isn't worth living are classic features of depression.

▶ WHAT YOU NEED TO KNOW

Depression is very common, affecting many people with and without diabetes worldwide. Unfortunately, persons with diabetes are twice as likely as others to have depression. It can be difficult to ask for help. The following six tips can help individuals feel more empowered to regain control of their lives:

TIP #1: WATCH FOR SIGNS OF DEPRESSION
Everyone feels sad every now and then. But how can you tell when sadness has turned into depression? People who are depressed will experience some of the following symptoms nearly every day for 2 weeks or more:
- Persistent "sad" mood
- Fatigue (loss of energy)
- Difficulty concentrating
- Irritability
- Feelings of guilt, hopelessness, or worthlessness
- Noticeable weight loss or gain
- Loss of appetite or binging on unhealthy foods
- Difficulty sleeping or sleeping more than usual
- Feeling restless
- Loss of interest or pleasure in usual activities
- Thoughts of suicide or hurting oneself

- Other bodily symptoms such as aches, pains, headaches, or digestive problems without a clear cause

TIP #2: DEPRESSION CAN MAKE DIABETES MANAGEMENT MORE DIFFICULT

People who are depressed feel less motivated to take care of themselves. As a result, they might exercise less, eat an unhealthy diet or fail to check their blood glucose or take their medications. All these factors can lead to potentially preventable complications from diabetes. Ask your health care provider for help—with proper treatment, you'll feel better inside and out.

TIP #3: TALK TO YOUR DOCTOR ABOUT DEPRESSION

People are sometimes taken by surprise when their health care provider expresses concerns about depression. Nonetheless, if you have trouble controlling your blood glucose levels despite your best efforts at a healthy lifestyle, consider whether your mood might be contributing. If you are depressed, your health care provider can help. Speak up!

TIP #4: DON'T SUFFER ALONE—HELP IS AVAILABLE

Two common treatment options are available for people who have depression: a talk therapy–based approach and a medication-based approach. Before prescribing drugs, a health care provider might encourage people to exercise, improve their diet, and work with a therapist to discover new ways of approaching challenges. If lifestyle changes and therapy aren't enough to improve mood, several effective medicines are available. Antidepressants are medicines that treat depression. They can help the brain more effectively use certain chemicals that control mood or stress. The most commonly prescribed family of medications is known as *selective serotonin reuptake inhibitors*, or simply SSRIs. This family includes citalopram (brand name Celexa), escitalopram (brand name Lexapro), paroxetine (brand name Paxil), sertraline (brand name Zoloft), and fluoxetine (brand name Prozac). Another common class of medications includes *serotonin and norepinephrine reuptake inhibitors* (SNRIs), such as venlafaxine (brand name Effexor), desvenlafaxine (brand name Pristiq), levomilnacipran (brand name Fetzima), and duloxetine (brand name Cymbalta). There are several other antidepressants, as well; talk to your health care provider about the best medication for you.

TIP #5: WAIT FOR IT—DEPRESSION MEDICINES DON'T WORK RIGHT AWAY

Some people feel discouraged and stop taking these medications when they don't notice immediate improvement. It's important to remember that these medicines normally take a few weeks to affect mood. If you begin to have thoughts of hurting or killing yourself, however, notify your health care provider immediately.

TIP #6: TELL YOUR PROVIDER ABOUT
UNPLEASANT SIDE EFFECTS

Each person will react differently to depression medications. Some drugs can upset the stomach, cause dry mouth, or worsen fatigue. Talk to your health care provider if this occurs; there are many other medications to try instead.

WHAT DOES IT ALL MEAN?

People with diabetes might not realize they also have depression, and many people are hesitant to ask for help. It is important to remember that depression is common, and there are many options available to improve a person's mood and increase the enjoyment of everyday life. This will improve mental health and help a person better manage her or his diabetes.

THE EYES
Retinopathy

While the entire eye is vulnerable to injury, one part in particular—the retina—is especially sensitive to damage in people with diabetes. The retina detects light and converts it to signals sent through the optic nerve to the brain. Damage to the retina from diabetes, known as *diabetic retinopathy*, is more common among people with chronically high blood glucose levels and persons who have had diabetes for many years.

▶ WHAT YOU NEED TO KNOW

The majority of people with type 1 diabetes—and many of those with type 2 diabetes—experience at least some degree of retinopathy after living with the disease for more than 10 to 20 years. Poorly managed blood glucose levels increase the risk of retinopathy, and infrequent visits to the eye specialist can delay diagnosis and lead to serious complications. Diabetic retinopathy is the number one cause of visual loss among people with diabetes and the leading cause of visual impairment and vision loss among working-age adults.

Retinopathy can be classified as nonproliferative or proliferative (figure 7.4). In *nonproliferative retinopathy*, small areas of balloon-like swelling in the retina's

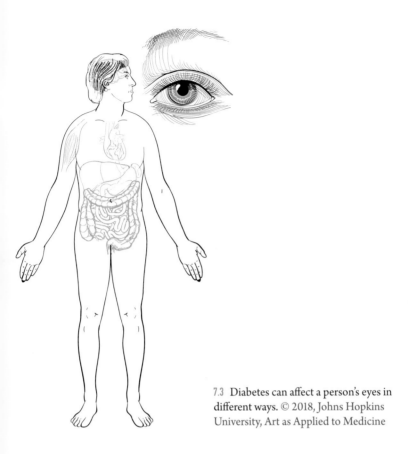

7.3 Diabetes can affect a person's eyes in different ways. © 2018, Johns Hopkins University, Art as Applied to Medicine

blood vessels, called *microaneurysms*, occur and may bleed (called *hemorrhages*) or leak fluid into the retina. This can lead to swelling in the retina. As nonproliferative retinopathy becomes more severe, parts of the retina may not receive an adequate blood supply. Your eye specialist, or ophthalmologist, may classify this further as mild, moderate, or severe disease, depending on the findings. In severe disease, called *proliferative diabetic retinopathy*, new abnormal blood vessels grow on the surface of the retina. These new vessels are very fragile and are more likely to leak and bleed, leading to sudden vision loss. The abnormal proliferation of blood vessels and scarring can then tug the retina and lead to a retinal detachment—the pulling away of the retina from underlying tissue—resulting in permanent vision loss.

Preventing Diabetic Retinopathy

People with diabetes can reduce their risk of retinopathy—and slow the progression of existing eye disease—by following these tips:

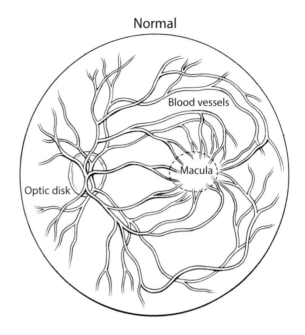

Normal

Blood vessels

Macula

Optic disk

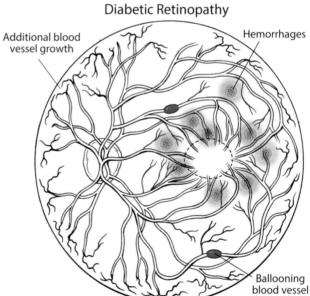

Diabetic Retinopathy

Additional blood vessel growth

Hemorrhages

Ballooning blood vessel

7.4 Multiple changes can be seen in diabetic retinopathy, including ballooning of the blood vessels in the eyes (*microaneurysms*), bleeding into the eye (*hemorrhages*), and additional blood vessel growth in the eyes. Diabetic retinopathy can lead to vision loss.
© 2018, Johns Hopkins University, Art as Applied to Medicine

- Maintain good blood glucose levels.
- Control high blood pressure and high cholesterol.
- Seek treatment for heart disease and kidney disease.
- Schedule yearly checkups with an eye specialist for a dilated eye exam; more frequent exams are needed if diagnosed with retinopathy.
- Women who are pregnant and have any stage of retinopathy will need to get their eyes examined more frequently since retinopathy can worsen during pregnancy.

Contact an ophthalmologist if any of the following symptoms develop:

- Seeing "flashes" of light
- Seeing spots or "floaters"
- Decreased or distorted vision
- Blurriness
- Fluctuations in vision quality
- Difficulty seeing at night
- Shadows or blind spots

Treatment Options

Mild to moderate diabetic retinopathy often benefits from careful monitoring and control of blood glucose levels under the close supervision of an eye doctor. Injections of medications into the eye and laser therapy are used to treat more severe retinopathy.

WHAT DOES IT ALL MEAN?

- Diabetic retinopathy can be prevented with good management of blood glucose, blood pressure, and cholesterol.
- Diabetic retinopathy can often go unnoticed until vision loss occurs—underscoring the importance of early detection, timely treatment, and appropriate follow-up.
- People with diabetes should have a comprehensive dilated eye exam at least once a year by an ophthalmologist or optometrist.

Cataracts

Cataract is a condition in which the eye's naturally clear lens becomes cloudy or opaque. Because light cannot pass as easily through the lens, it is not properly reflected onto the retina, resulting in vision being cloudy or blurry. In people with diabetes, high blood glucose levels can cause the lens to swell, and this can affect the structure of naturally occurring proteins. These changes contribute to cataract formation and put people with diabetes at higher risk of developing them.

▶ WHAT YOU NEED TO KNOW

What Are the Symptoms?

- Cloudy or blurry vision
- Decreased vision with bright lights (for example, glare from oncoming headlights or bright sunlight)
- Seeing halos around lights
- Poor night vision
- Seeing dull, rather than vibrant, colors
- Seeing multiple images in one eye

Cataracts usually develop in both eyes but might become worse in one eye.

How Are Cataracts Treated?

- Prescription eye glasses and brighter lighting will sometimes improve vision for people with early or mild cataracts.
- Surgery is sometimes performed to treat advanced cataracts that prevent people from completing their normal daily activities.
- Talk to your health care provider about treating any other diabetic eye diseases *before* undergoing cataract surgery, as the timing of these procedures can affect the overall health of the eyes.

What Are the Risks with Diabetes?

- People with type 1 and type 2 diabetes are more likely than others to develop cataracts and typically do so at a younger age.

WHAT DOES IT ALL M EAN?

People with diabetes should be screened regularly for eye conditions, including cataracts. If a person with diabetes has both cataracts and diabetic eye disease, such as retinopathy, the diabetic eye disease is usually treated first, before the person undergoes cataract surgery.

Macular Edema

The macula is a small but important area in the center of the retina that allows you to clearly see the details of objects right in front of you. *Macular edema* is a condition that occurs when blood vessels in the eye leak fluid and protein into the macula, resulting in swelling and blurred vision. It occurs more commonly in those with diabetes.

▶ WHAT YOU NEED TO KNOW

Macular edema affects many people with diabetes. This condition causes vision in one or both eyes to become blurry, usually in the area of central vision. Macular edema can occur with both nonproliferative and proliferative retinopathy.

Diagnosis

Reporting persistently blurry vision to your health care provider is very important. You may be referred to an ophthalmologist for a dilated eye exam. The ophthalmologist will be able to check for changes in the retina, such as macular edema, which could be affecting your vision.

Treatment

Leaky blood vessels can be repaired using lasers or by injecting medications that slow the growth of new blood vessels. These medications are part of a relatively new treatment strategy called *intravitreal anti-VEGF therapy*; more than one injection is usually required. Your eye specialist might also prescribe anti-inflammatory or steroid eye drops.

Following treatment, the ophthalmologist will need to keep close track of your eyes to prevent further damage. You may be asked to return for a follow-up exam every 2 to 4 months to make sure your eyes recover properly.

WHAT DOES IT ALL MEAN?

- Macular edema is a condition that starts with blurred vision but can lead to blindness.
- It is much more common among with those with diabetes.
- Managing your glucose well will help prevent or reduce your chances of macular edema.
- Diagnosis requires referral to an eye specialist, and several treatment options exist.
- Early treatment of macular edema can halt or even reverse vision loss.
- Close follow-up is needed to ensure a full recovery.

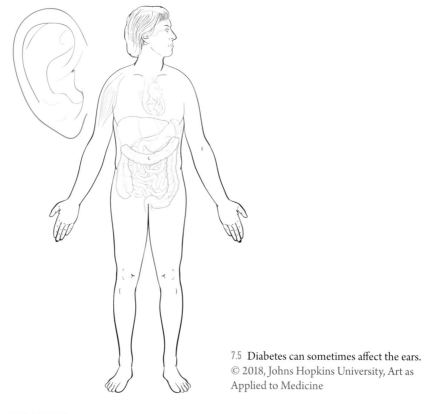

7.5 Diabetes can sometimes affect the ears. © 2018, Johns Hopkins University, Art as Applied to Medicine

THE EARS

Hearing Loss

People with diabetes are at increased risk of *sensorineural hearing loss,* which occurs when the ear has trouble sending information from sounds along the auditory nerve to the brain.

▶ WHAT YOU NEED TO KNOW

Hearing loss can begin with a subtle warning sign—trouble following a conversation in a crowded room or a nagging feeling that everyone around you is mumbling—but over a period of years, the signs of hearing loss become more obvious.

Most people think of hearing loss as a condition of older people or of musicians who like their music loud. But you might be surprised to learn that hearing loss is also common among smokers, people who take certain medications, and—you guessed it—people with diabetes. In fact, hearing loss is up to twice as common in people with diabetes than in people without diabetes.

What Are the Symptoms of Hearing Loss?

During the early stages of sensorineural hearing loss, a person finds it difficult to detect high frequency sounds, such as a small metal triangle clanging against a rod. As the disease progresses, lower frequencies—such as a bass drum—might become a problem as well. Over time, the hearing loss will become more noticeable.

How Is Hearing Loss Diagnosed?

If your family suspects you have hearing loss, or if you've noticed the symptoms yourself, your health care provider might perform a number of tests to measure your hearing. One of the tests will determine if you can hear and understand a whispered voice. Another test might check your ability to tell whether a tuning fork is louder in one ear than another. The provider might refer you to an ear, nose, and throat doctor, along with a specialist known as an *audiologist*. These specialists will check your inner and middle ears and potentially recommend hearing aids or other assistive devices.

Are There Any Treatments for Hearing Loss Other Than Hearing Aids?

Hearing aids remain the main treatment for sensorineural hearing loss. If you have hearing loss, talk to your health care provider and pharmacist about avoiding certain medications known to damage the ears as a side effect.

WHAT DOES IT ALL MEAN?

Hearing loss is more common in people with diabetes. If hearing loss is suspected, visiting a specialist and considering the need for a hearing aid can be useful.

THE MOUTH
Tooth and Gum Disease

Periodontal disease refers to problems with the teeth and gums. This can lead to the loss of teeth and may be associated with cardiovascular disease. People with diabetes are more likely to have gum disease and tooth decay.

▶ WHAT YOU NEED TO KNOW

Dental health is much more than bright teeth and fresh breath. Taking care of your mouth, including your gums, teeth, tongue, and cheeks, can improve over-

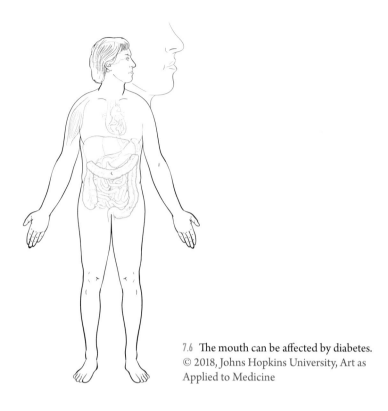

7.6 The mouth can be affected by diabetes.
© 2018, Johns Hopkins University, Art as
Applied to Medicine

all wellness by preventing infection, keeping blood sugar in check, and even promoting a healthy heart.

Many people struggle with dental care. Many adults can develop swollen, inflamed gums with infected pockets surrounding each tooth. This condition, periodontal disease, can lead to the loss of teeth. Some studies have shown that periodontal disease can increase the risk of heart attack and stroke. Unfortunately, periodontal disease is much more common in people with diabetes than in the general public. This risk is even higher for cigarette smokers.

How Does This Happen?

The human mouth normally contains many types of bacteria. A number of these bacteria are helpful, but some cause bad breath and tooth decay. The balance of the good versus bad bacteria is important. When bad bacteria outnumber the good, it can lead to periodontal disease. Factors that can increase this risk include eating a high-sugar diet, failing to brush and floss regularly, and having an underlying health condition such as diabetes.

Some people with diabetes have an especially high risk of periodontal disease:

- Pregnant or menopausal women
- Older persons
- Immunosuppressed people, including those with leukemia, HIV or AIDS, or those undergoing chemotherapy
- Smokers and substance abusers

The body fights off this infection by mounting an immune response. But the inflammation from this immune response can often further damage the teeth.

How Will I Know If I Have This Condition?

Tell your health care provider if you notice any of these symptoms:
- Swollen, sore gums that bleed easily during brushing and flossing
- Lingering bad breath and an unpleasant taste in the mouth
- Loose teeth or a newly formed gap between your teeth
- A blister, or fluid pocket, on the gum tissue, especially if teeth in the surrounding area are tender
- Any of these symptoms accompanied by unusual increases in blood glucose levels

Your provider will refer you to a dentist, who can perform an oral exam and take x-rays to check for signs of bone loss near the tooth socket.

How Is It Treated?

The treatment of periodontal disease often begins with a dental deep cleaning, where the dentist removes plaque from the affected teeth and roots. Some people are encouraged to use an antimicrobial mouthwash to prevent the build-up of bad bacteria on and between teeth. More serious cases might require minor surgery to remove diseased tissue or treat an abscess, as well as antibiotics to treat an infection.

After treatment, people with diabetes are encouraged to schedule a follow-up exam in 3 to 4 months to check for signs of improvement. Treating periodontal disease usually also helps blood glucose management, making diabetes more manageable.

WHAT DOES IT ALL MEAN?

- Periodontal disease refers to inflammation around the gums, which can result in loss of teeth.
- People with diabetes are at increased risk of periodontal disease.
- Regular teeth brushing, flossing, and trips to the dentist can help prevent periodontal disease.

THE THYROID
Thyroid Disease

That small gland at the base of your neck, known as the *thyroid*, plays an enormous role in everyday health. The thyroid makes hormones that control how fast you burn calories and how fast your heart beats, among other vital functions.

If this gland malfunctions, too much or too little thyroid hormone can be delivered to the body. A shortage of hormone is known as *hypothyroidism* and is the most common type of thyroid disease in people with diabetes. The excessive production of hormone is known as *hyperthyroidism*.

Many women with type 2 diabetes have hypothyroidism, but it is unclear if these two conditions are truly linked or just occur together because they are both common in the general population. It's less common in men but can occur in people of either sex who become resistant to insulin, as occurs in type 2 diabetes. And 15% to 30% of people with type 1 diabetes will have thyroid disease caused by autoimmunity.

▶ WHAT YOU NEED TO KNOW

What Are the Symptoms and Signs of Thyroid Disease?

Hypothyroidism (underactive thyroid) can cause the following symptoms:
- Fatigue
- Weight gain (without eating more)
- Sensitivity to cold temperatures
- Constipation
- Dry skin
- Muscle pain
- Menstrual irregularities
- Slow heart rate (less than 60 beats per minute)
- Swelling and fluid retention in the hands, feet, or legs
- Changes in blood glucose levels and a change in insulin needs

Hyperthyroidism (overactive thyroid) can cause the following symptoms:
- Weight loss (even with eating more)
- Sensitivity to hot temperatures
- Excessive sweating
- Tremor
- Hard, fast, or irregular heartbeat (palpitations)
- High blood pressure (especially systolic, the top number)

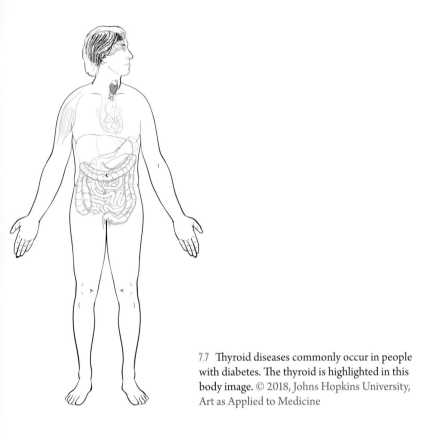

7.7 Thyroid diseases commonly occur in people with diabetes. The thyroid is highlighted in this body image. © 2018, Johns Hopkins University, Art as Applied to Medicine

- Anxiety, hyperactivity, or temperamental mood swings
- Increased number of bowel movements
- Muscle weakness and exaggerated reflexes
- Menstrual irregularities
- Swelling of the breast tissue or erectile dysfunction in some men
- Elevation of glucose levels and increased need for insulin

How Is Thyroid Disease Diagnosed and Treated?

If you have diabetes, it's especially important to let your provider know if you experience any of the symptoms and signs described previously. Your provider will examine your neck and perform a blood test to measure *thyroid-stimulating hormone (TSH)* levels and sometimes the free T4 and T3 levels as well. The provider may also check for antibodies in the blood, which could indicate you have an autoimmune disease, and your immune system is mistakenly attacking your own thyroid.

You might require routine screening for thyroid problems if

- you were recently told you have type 1 diabetes,
- you've had a baby within the past year and have type 1 diabetes,
- you have eye changes suggesting a related autoimmune condition, such as Graves' orbitopathy.

The treatment and follow-up for people with thyroid disease will follow the same treatment used for people without diabetes.

WHAT DOES IT ALL MEAN?

- Thyroid disease is common in people with diabetes.
- The most common thyroid disorder is hypothyroidism (an underactive thyroid), which can be treated with a daily thyroid hormone replacement pill.
- People with type 1 diabetes are more likely to develop other autoimmune conditions, such as thyroid disease, and need testing as described.

THE HEART AND RELATED CONDITIONS (HYPERTENSION AND DYSLIPIDEMIA)

Diagnosing and Managing Heart Disease

The terms *macrovascular disease* and *cardiovascular disease* refer to narrowing in any of the large blood vessels of the body, such as those leading to the heart, brain, and legs, mainly due to a buildup of fatty deposits (or *plaque*) in the arteries. A myocardial infarction (or "heart attack") results when blood supplying the heart itself is suddenly slowed or stopped because of an extremely narrowed or blocked blood vessel (figure 7.9).

▶ WHAT YOU NEED TO KNOW

In general, persons with diabetes are two to four times as likely as others to develop heart disease. It is the leading cause of death in people with diabetes. In addition, people with diabetes usually develop heart disease at a younger age than those without diabetes, so early prevention is critical.

Over time, high blood glucose levels can damage large and small blood vessels that lead to your heart, brain, legs, nerves, kidneys, and other parts of the body. The longer you have diabetes, the more likely you are to develop heart disease.

What Are the Risk Factors for Heart Disease?

A family history of early heart disease and older age are strong risk factors

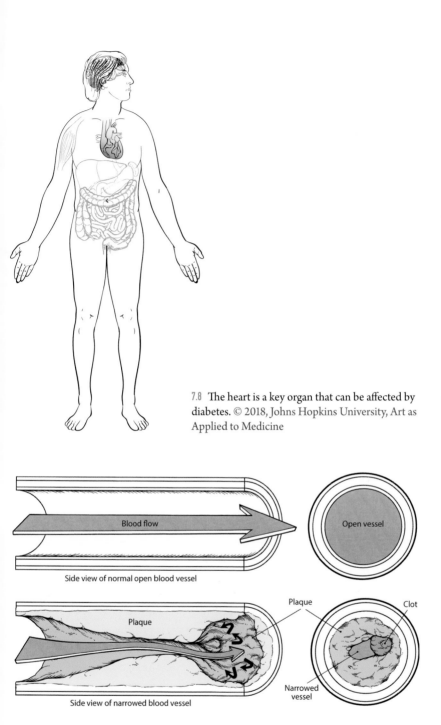

7.8 The heart is a key organ that can be affected by diabetes. © 2018, Johns Hopkins University, Art as Applied to Medicine

Blood flow

Open vessel

Side view of normal open blood vessel

Plaque

Plaque

Clot

Narrowed vessel

Side view of narrowed blood vessel

7.9 A comparison of a normal blood vessel with one narrowed by plaque in a person with cardiovascular disease. © 2018, Johns Hopkins University, Art as Applied to Medicine

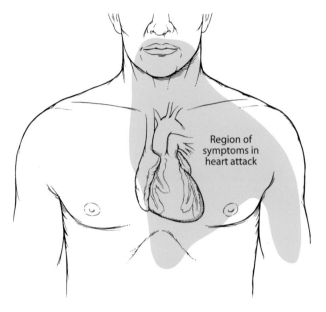

Region of
symptoms in
heart attack

7.10 Locations where pain can occur with angina or a heart attack. © 2018, Johns Hopkins University, Art as Applied to Medicine

for cardiovascular disease. Other common risk factors include smoking, high blood pressure, abnormal cholesterol levels (high LDL, or bad cholesterol; low HDL, or good cholesterol; and high triglycerides), obesity, and physical inactivity. People with diabetes and poorly managed blood glucose levels are also at a higher risk of developing cardiovascular disease. Young men with erectile dysfunction and people with diabetes who have kidney disease are also more likely to have cardiovascular disease and should be assessed for other risk factors.

Warning Signs

Because these symptoms could be signs of a heart attack, seek urgent medical attention if you experience

- chest discomfort when you walk or exercise that lasts longer than a few minutes or comes back repeatedly (also called *angina*);
- chest pain accompanied by fatigue or shortness of breath, sweating, light-headedness, or nausea;
- pain or discomfort with exercise in one or both of your arms or shoulders or your upper or mid-back, neck, or jaw (figure 7.10).

Sometimes a heart attack can occur with no obvious symptoms and without a person knowing it. This is called a *silent heart attack*. Silent heart attacks are more common in persons with diabetes. Diabetes-related nerve damage that blunts chest pain may be one reason why symptoms aren't always noticed. Regular medical checkups are key in persons with diabetes. Early treatment can reduce or delay cardiovascular disease.

How Is Heart Disease Detected?

Health care providers use a variety of tests to detect heart disease. An electrocardiogram (EKG) can reveal whether the heart's electrical activity is normal. A stress test on a treadmill can provide further information. If you are not able to walk on a treadmill, your provider may "stress" your heart by injecting medications through an intravenous (IV) infusion. This medicine can cause the heart to beat faster and mimic the stress of exercise. Some patients may have an echocardiogram or a nuclear medicine heart scan, which provides pictures of the heart to reveal how well its muscles pump blood. Other blood tests may be performed in the emergency room to diagnose a heart attack.

WHAT DOES IT ALL MEAN?

Reduce your risk of cardiovascular disease today by making the following changes. Ask your provider to help you

- quit smoking;
- lose weight;
- manage stress;
- eat a healthy diet (see "Dietary Therapy" on page 83);
- exercise regularly (see "Physical Activity and Exercise" on page 95);
- control your blood pressure (see "Managing Hypertension" on page 129);
- improve your cholesterol levels (see "Managing Dyslipidemia" on page 131);
- set an appropriate A1C target with your provider and work toward that goal; and
- take medications as appropriate, such as aspirin or statins, to reduce your risk of heart disease. If you have had a heart attack in the past, your provider may recommend specific medications to treat diabetes that have also been found to reduce the risk of having another heart attack.

Congestive Heart Failure

Congestive heart failure (sometimes referred to as CHF or simply "heart failure") is a common disorder as people age. This occurs more often in patients with diabetes. *Systolic heart failure* means that the heart is not pumping blood as well as it should. *Diastolic heart failure* means that the heart has trouble relaxing and allowing blood to flow into its chambers between beats. This occurs when the walls of the heart become stiff.

▶ WHAT YOU NEED TO KNOW

Key Facts about Heart Failure

1 Heart failure means that the heart is no longer able to pump enough blood to meet the needs of the body. People with heart failure have an increased risk of sudden death.

2 The risk of heart failure rises dramatically with age. In fact, it's one of the most common reasons for hospitalization in adults older than 75.

3 People with diabetes are much more likely than others to develop heart failure. Many of the risk factors that go along with diabetes, such as high blood pressure and coronary artery disease, are also risk factors for heart failure.

4 Coronary artery disease is a leading cause of heart failure. When a coronary artery (vessels that supply blood to the heart) is blocked, this can lead to heart muscle damage. This may result in the heart no longer pumping blood as well as it should.

5 Heart failure leads to the buildup of fluid in the body, known as *edema.* If fluid accumulates in the lungs, it can also lead to a lingering cough, shortness of breath, and fatigue. Many people have trouble breathing when they lie flat on their backs. Other symptoms include swollen legs, weakness, weight gain, and an enlarged or bloated belly.

6 If you have symptoms of heart failure, your provider will perform a number of tests before you are diagnosed with the condition. An EKG can often be performed in the medical provider's office to determine if you have had a heart attack and if your heart rhythm is normal. Your provider might also recommend a chest x-ray to get a better idea of the amount of congestion in your lungs and the size and shape of your heart. A test known as an echocardiogram will measure how well the walls of your heart are pumping and relaxing, while a cardiac angiogram can reveal any blockages or damage to the coronary arteries of the heart.

7 Heart failure is a serious condition, but several treatments can help. People with a history of heart failure should avoid salty foods or adding extra salt to their food. Providers often prescribe medications such as diuretics or "fluid pills" (see "Diuretics" on page 276) to help with the symptoms of heart failure by eliminating excess fluid accumulation. Blood pressure medications such as angiotensin-converting enzyme (ACE) inhibitors,

angiotensin-receptor blockers (ARBs), and beta-blockers are often used for the long-term treatment of heart failure (see "Medications for High Blood Pressure" on page 269). Other medications, including cholesterol medications (such as statins), may also be prescribed. People who are hospitalized, however, are often treated with oxygen and IV diuretics to remove excess fluids from the body.

8 Some diabetes drugs should not be taken by people with heart failure. Medications known as *thiazolidinediones* (pioglitazone or rosiglitazone; see "Thiazolidinediones" on page 242) can increase the risk of developing heart failure, worsen existing heart failure, and lead people to retain even more fluid. These medications should be avoided in those who have symptoms from heart failure or have more advanced stages of heart failure. People with diabetes and heart failure may be at increased risk of a condition that leads to the buildup of acid in blood, called *lactic acidosis*, when taking metformin.

9 If you have heart failure, work with your provider to set specific treatment goals. If you have systolic heart failure, for example, your goal might be to have normal electrolyte levels, a slow resting heart rate, good blood pressure (see "Managing Hypertension" on this page), and a healthy body weight. People with heart failure are best treated by a team of medical experts who work together and communicate often. Your team may include a heart doctor (*cardiologist*), a diabetes specialist (*endocrinologist*), and an internal medicine specialist in addition to nurse practitioners, dietitians, and pharmacists.

WHAT DOES IT ALL MEAN?

Heart failure occurs when the heart is not able to pump blood throughout the body as it should. This typically leads to fluid buildup or edema. People with diabetes are at higher risk for heart failure. Treating high blood pressure and preventing coronary artery disease are ways to lower the risk for heart failure.

Managing Hypertension

More than half of all persons with diabetes have a condition called *hypertension*, defined as a blood pressure higher than 140/90 millimeters of mercury (mmHg). The top number is called the *systolic* blood pressure and is the highest blood pressure your heart muscle exerts when pumping blood out during a heartbeat (or during the heart's contraction phase), while the bottom number is called the *diastolic* blood pressure and represents the lowest pressure in the arteries between heartbeats (or during the heart's relaxation phase).

▶ WHAT YOU NEED TO KNOW

Many health care providers believe that controlling blood pressure is at least as important, or even more important, as controlling blood glucose levels to prevent cardiovascular disease. Left untreated, high blood pressure levels can lead to heart disease, stroke, and even early death and further increase the risk of eye disease and kidney complications in persons with diabetes.

The factors related to high blood pressure may differ for each type of diabetes. High blood pressure is more common in persons with type 2 diabetes who are also obese. In persons with type 1 diabetes, high blood pressure tends to be more common in those with kidney disease.

High blood pressure often goes undetected because most people don't have symptoms. When symptoms of high blood pressure do occur, they might include headaches, chest pain, shortness of breath, or blurred vision.

In people with diabetes, the blood pressure goal is usually less than 140/90 mmHg, but this may be individualized. For instance, a lower goal (less than 130/80 mmHg) may be recommended if you are at higher risk of developing cardiovascular disease. Talk to your health care provider about the blood pressure goal that is appropriate for you.

Tips to Prevent the Progression to Hypertension
Lifestyle Changes:
- Reduce salt (sodium) intake.
- Meet with a dietitian to develop a DASH- (Dietary Approaches to Stop Hypertension) style diet, which has been shown to effectively lower high blood pressure. The DASH diet is high in fruits, vegetables, and low-fat or nonfat dairy. The DASH diet emphasizes whole grains and is rich in potassium, magnesium, calcium, and fiber.
- Moderate your alcohol intake (no more than one to two drinks per day).
- Exercise regularly (150 minutes per week).
- Achieve a weight loss goal of 5% to 7%.
- Stop smoking.
- Manage stress.

Medications:
- Medications such as ACE inhibitors, ARBs, some calcium channel

blockers, or thiazide-like diuretics have been shown to reduce the risk of cardiovascular disease in persons with diabetes if blood pressure doesn't improve after lifestyle changes or if blood pressure levels are very high at diagnosis (see "Medications for High Blood Pressure" on page 269).

- In people with diabetes and hypertension who also have albuminuria (see "Testing for Albuminuria" on page 156), ACE inhibitors and ARBs are often preferred.

WHAT DOES IT ALL MEAN?

People with diabetes are at risk for developing hypertension and often do not have any symptoms. Left untreated, high blood pressure can lead to heart attacks, strokes, and even premature death and increases the risk of eye disease and kidney complications. Check your blood pressure at home if it has been high in the past and at every doctor's visit. There are many preventive steps that if taken now may reduce your chance of developing hypertension in the future.

Managing Dyslipidemia

Have you ever been told that you have "bad" or "unhealthy" cholesterol levels? If so, your health care provider might have used the term *dyslipidemia* to describe your condition. Dyslipidemia covers more than just high levels of "bad" cholesterol (LDL), however. It also describes an excess of triglycerides—components of fats and oils—and lower levels of "good" cholesterol (HDL) in your blood. Over time, dyslipidemia is present in more than half of persons with diabetes. Dyslipidemia is a major risk factor for cardiovascular disease.

▶ WHAT YOU NEED TO KNOW

A person with dyslipidemia has abnormal levels of lipids, such as cholesterol and triglycerides, in the blood.

Cholesterol comes in many forms:

- HDL is known as "good" cholesterol. Women with diabetes should keep their HDL levels above 50 milligrams per deciliter (mg/dL); men above 40 mg/dL.
- LDL is known as "bad" cholesterol. Statin medications in particular can help lower LDL levels and prevent heart disease, stroke, and peripheral vascular disease.

Triglycerides are components of fats and oils:

- High fasting triglyceride levels are commonly considered to be above 150 mg/dL.
- Levels higher than 500 mg/dL at any time of day are considered dangerously high.

Persons with dyslipidemia and type 2 diabetes often have the worst of every category: not enough good cholesterol, too much bad cholesterol, and high levels of triglycerides.

How Is Dyslipidemia Treated?

Treatment always begins with healthy lifestyle changes. If you have dyslipidemia, your health care provider might arrange for you to meet with a dietitian.

In the meantime, follow these simple tips for improving your cholesterol:

- Start by looking at the nutritional facts on your food packaging.
- Reduce saturated and trans unsaturated fat intake and increase omega-3 fatty acids and viscous fiber (such as in oats, legumes, flax, beans, and citrus) in your diet.
- Exercising, losing weight, quitting smoking, and controlling blood glucose levels will help.
- If healthy lifestyle changes aren't enough, your health care provider might recommend oral medications to improve your lipid levels, such as statins, ezetimibe, niacin, omega-3 fatty acids, fibrates, or bile acid sequestrants. In addition, PCSK9 inhibitors are a relatively newer class of injectable lipid-lowering medications that may sometimes be used to lower LDL levels in persons with a history of heart disease or stroke, in persons who are intolerant to statins, or in combination with statins, if cholesterol goals are not met (see "Medications for Cholesterol Abnormalities" on page 277).
- Generally, all persons with diabetes who are 40 years and older should be on statin medications because they can effectively lower the risk of premature death, heart attack, stroke, and peripheral vascular disease, even among those without dyslipidemia or a history of macrovascular disease. Talk to your health care provider to see if this class of medications might be beneficial for you.

WHAT DOES IT ALL MEAN?

Dyslipidemia greatly increases your risk of complications from diabetes, including heart attack, stroke, and peripheral vascular disease, particularly as you get older. Early detection of dyslipidemia through regular cholesterol screenings and statin treatment is essential to preventing complications. Statin medications not only lower LDL cholesterol levels effectively but also prevent heart disease in people with diabetes. Most people with diabetes should be taking a statin medication; talk to your provider to see if one is appropriate for you.

Managing Metabolic Syndrome

Metabolic syndrome refers to a group or cluster of related health conditions, including obesity, high blood pressure, cholesterol abnormalities, and prediabetes or diabetes that often occur together and can increase your risk for heart disease.

▶ WHAT YOU NEED TO KNOW

Facts about Metabolic Syndrome

1 When a provider says a person has metabolic syndrome, it indicates that the person has multiple health conditions (usually three or more) that together pose a serious risk for heart disease, diabetes, or both. These conditions might include the following:
   - ✓ A large waistline (central obesity), such as a waist circumference over 40 inches (102 centimeters) in men or 35 inches (88 centimeters) in women; these cutoffs vary for people of different ethnicities
   - ✓ Blood pressure 130/85 mmHg or higher (prehypertension or hypertension)
   - ✓ Blood glucose 100 mg/dL or 5.6 millimoles per liter (mmol/L) or higher after fasting for 8 hours (prediabetes or diabetes)
   - ✓ Elevated triglycerides after fasting for 8 hours (150 mg/dL or higher)
   - ✓ Low amounts of good HDL cholesterol (less than 50 mg/dL for women; less than 40 mg/dL for men)
2 Metabolic syndrome is a common condition and is referred to by many different names (*syndrome X* or *insulin resistance syndrome*).
3 Metabolic syndrome is usually diagnosed in people who are overweight or obese. These people are more likely than others to have high blood pressure, type 2 diabetes, and high levels of triglycerides in their blood.
4 If you've been diagnosed with metabolic syndrome, you're not alone: one in every three U.S. adults has this condition! Your chances of developing metabolic syndrome increase with age.
5 People with metabolic syndrome are three to four times more likely than oth-

ers to develop type 2 diabetes. Also, having diabetes *and* metabolic syndrome dramatically increases your chances of developing heart disease and stroke.

6 Most people with metabolic syndrome can be treated with these positive lifestyle changes:

  ✓ Losing body weight of 5% to 7%
  ✓ Eating a healthy, balanced diet
  ✓ Exercising at least 150 minutes a week
  ✓ Quitting smoking

7 Sometimes, lifestyle changes aren't enough to manage metabolic syndrome. If the condition doesn't improve despite a person's best efforts, providers might treat each component of metabolic syndrome separately. The treatment plan might include medications to lower blood pressure, improve cholesterol, or regulate blood glucose.

WHAT DOES IT ALL MEAN?

Metabolic syndrome represents a series of abnormalities that together increase the risk for diabetes and heart disease. Weight loss, exercise, and diet changes can help lower the risk of metabolic syndrome progressing to diabetes and heart disease. Metabolic syndrome is important to identify early.

THE CIRCULATION

Peripheral Arterial Disease

Peripheral vascular disease occurs when a blood vessel in a location other than the brain or heart becomes abnormally narrowed or blocked. This can occur either in the arteries or veins. *Peripheral artery disease* (PAD) is a type of peripheral vascular disease caused by fatty buildups (atherosclerosis) in the inner walls of arteries. This blockage prevents blood from circulating normally throughout the body, usually to the legs or feet, resulting in pain or fatigue, especially during walking. The pain usually improves with rest.

▶ WHAT YOU NEED TO KNOW

People with diabetes are much more likely than people without diabetes to develop this condition. If you smoke, you're at an even higher risk. If you notice pain in your legs (calf muscles) or feet when you're walking that eases as soon as you rest, ask your health care provider if you should be tested for peripheral arterial disease.

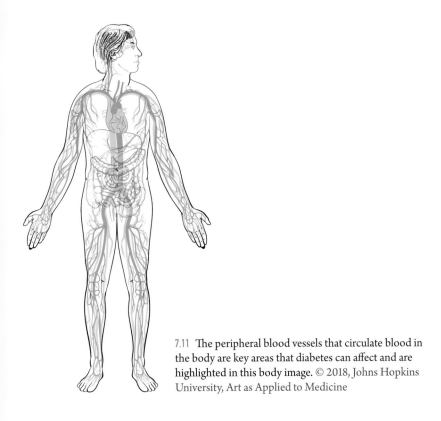

7.11 The peripheral blood vessels that circulate blood in the body are key areas that diabetes can affect and are highlighted in this body image. © 2018, Johns Hopkins University, Art as Applied to Medicine

Painful legs, particularly in the calves, with walking is also known as *claudication*. The pain you feel in your legs results from a narrowed artery reducing blood flow to your muscles and limiting the oxygen and nutrients delivered to them. Since the muscles need more oxygen during exercise, pain comes at that time. By itself, claudication is not worthy of an emergency room visit as long as your legs stop hurting when you rest. However, it is a warning sign of peripheral arterial disease—and it is very important to diagnose and treat this condition as quickly as possible (figure 7.12). Left untreated, claudication can become so severe that the pain no longer fades away when you rest. If this happens, call your health care provider right away. This could signal a near-complete block of blood flow known as *critical leg ischemia*. Other symptoms include foot sores or wounds that heal slowly, cold feet or bluish discoloration, and erectile dysfunction in men.

Warning!

Critical leg ischemia is a medical emergency and must be treated as soon as possible. Caught early, this condition can be treated surgically to restore blood

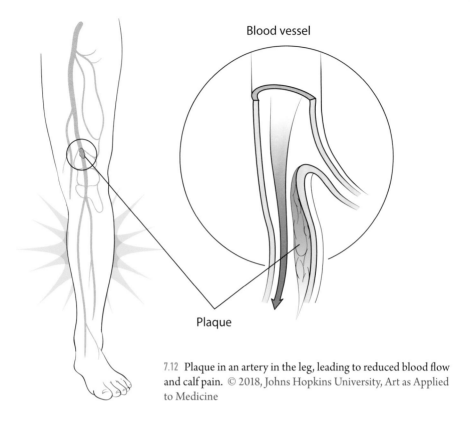

Blood vessel

Plaque

7.12 Plaque in an artery in the leg, leading to reduced blood flow and calf pain. © 2018, Johns Hopkins University, Art as Applied to Medicine

flow. But in severe cases, providers must remove, or amputate, the affected foot or leg. Always call your provider when you first notice symptoms of leg discomfort, particularly during exercise, even if they seem minor.

How Is Peripheral Vascular Disease Diagnosed?

Health care providers will usually ask a person with diabetes a list of questions to find out how long the pain has been present, what triggers it, and what it feels like. People with claudication usually notice that they can walk a specific distance or number of steps each time before they start to feel pain in their legs. This information helps providers distinguish claudication from other types of leg pain.

Certain imaging tests, like ultrasounds or angiograms, can detect blocked blood vessels. The provider might also measure the patient's blood pressure in the ankle and arm (*ankle brachial index*, or ABI) to make sure the results are similar. Lower blood pressure in the ankle compared with the arm might lead the doctor to suspect a blockage in blood flow to the legs.

How Is It Treated?

Depending on how severe your condition is, your health care provider might recommend treatment ranging from lifestyle changes to surgery. A proper treatment plan could include any of the following suggestions:

- Quit smoking immediately. Smoking is one of the most important risk factors for PAD.
- Change your diet (see "Dietary Therapy" on page 83).
- Get regular exercise, including leg and foot calisthenics (see "Exercise" on page 95).
- Remember to check your feet every day for injuries, a change in color, or skin breakdown.
- Take blood pressure medications (see "Medications for High Blood Pressure" on page 269).
- Take cholesterol medications (see "Medications for Cholesterol Abnormalities" on page 277).
- Take medications to reduce blood clotting (see "Anticoagulants" and "Antiplatelet Medications" on pages 287).
- Have surgery to clear or bypass a blocked blood vessel.
- Don't walk barefoot.

WHAT DOES IT ALL MEAN?

Persons with diabetes who have a history of smoking, heart disease, stroke, or high blood pressure are at higher risk for peripheral vascular disease. Peripheral arterial disease can cause leg pain with walking that improves with rest. Treatments include lifestyle changes, medicines, and sometimes surgery. Proper foot care is important, including the avoidance of barefoot walking and checking feet regularly for signs of injury.

THE LUNGS AND BREATHING
Obstructive Sleep Apnea

People with diabetes who struggle with their weight—especially those who snore loudly at night—may occasionally stop breathing for short periods of time during their sleep. This is a condition called *obstructive sleep apnea* that can affect many people with diabetes.

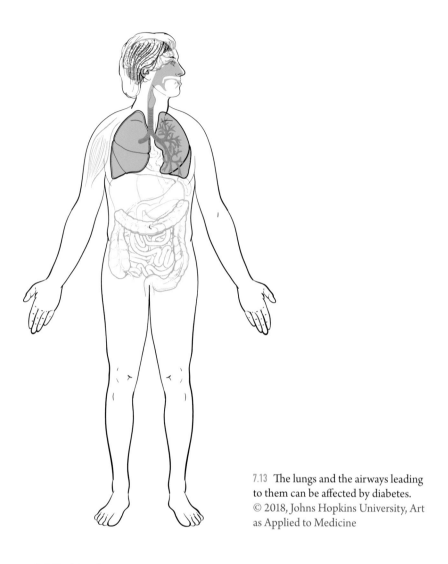

7.13 The lungs and the airways leading to them can be affected by diabetes.
© 2018, Johns Hopkins University, Art as Applied to Medicine

▶ WHAT YOU NEED TO KNOW

What Causes Obstructive Sleep Apnea?

Obesity is an important factor contributing to obstructive sleep apnea. Extra skin, fat, and muscle around the neck area lead to excess pressure against the airway and cause it to collapse when the person is lying down. When the airway collapses, the person stops breathing, typically only for a few seconds but for longer as the condition worsens. The person then has short awakenings (that he or she usually does not remember) and resumes breathing. While people do not remember these incidents, the repeated awakenings prevent restful sleep.

Because obesity and type 2 diabetes are often present together, it is common for people with type 2 diabetes to experience obstructive sleep apnea.

Should I Be Tested for Sleep Apnea?

People with type 2 diabetes who have symptoms such as snoring or daytime sleepiness should be tested for sleep apnea. The test can be done overnight in a sleep lab or even in the comfort of their own home. The test involves monitoring sleep with equipment to determine if a person stops breathing during the night.

If you answer yes to any of the following questions, ask your physician if you should be tested for sleep apnea:

- Are you overweight or obese?
- Do you have a thick neck (more than 16 inches around for women and 17 inches for men)?
- Do you snore heavily, especially with long pauses between each snore?
- Do you often startle in your sleep and wake up suddenly without knowing why?
- Do you occasionally gasp or choke during sleep?
- Are you exhausted in the morning, even after 8 or more hours of sleep?
- Do you have trouble concentrating or fall asleep easily during the day?

The Importance of Seeking Treatment

Many people who experience sleep apnea have high blood pressure and notice that their blood glucose levels are difficult to control. Heart disease can also develop more commonly in people who have both sleep apnea and diabetes.

Treatment may improve blood glucose control, lower blood pressure, and possibly improve cardiovascular health (table 7.1).

Important note: People treated for sleep apnea with positive airway pressure (PAP) should tell their providers if they gain or lose weight because the machine's settings may need to be adjusted. A repeat sleep test may reveal that PAP is no longer needed for some patients after weight loss.

WHAT DOES IT ALL MEAN?

- People with diabetes, especially those with obesity and type 2 diabetes, have a higher risk of sleep apnea than other people.
- Treatment of sleep apnea can help improve cardiovascular health.
- Weight loss is the most effective and least expensive treatment; other options include machines that deliver PAP through the mouth or nose at night.

Table 7.1. Treatment options for people with sleep apnea

OPTION	HOW IT WORKS	PROS	CONS
Weight loss	Less fat makes it less likely that the airway will collapse	Losing just 10% of body weight can improve, or in some cases cure, sleep apnea	It involves hard work by the person wishing to lose weight
PAP	PAP stands for positive airway pressure; it is a machine that pressurizes and humidifies air and delivers it to the body through a mask worn during sleep to prevent the airway from collapsing	It reduces blood pressure, may help control blood glucose, and prevents episodes of apnea	Some people find it difficult to fall asleep because of the mask, air blowing into the nose, or the sound of the machine
Mouth guards	These appliances fit in the mouth and keep the jaw in a position that supports an open airway	A good alternative if PAP is not an option	Many people find these devices uncomfortable, and insurance may not cover the costs
Surgery	Surgery is performed to open the upper airway	A good alternative if PAP is not an option	Invasive. Requires general anesthesia; recovery time and outcomes may not be as good

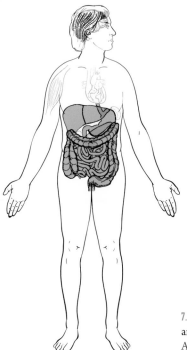

7.14 Diabetes can affect the stomach, liver, pancreas, and gut. © 2018, Johns Hopkins University, Art as Applied to Medicine

THE STOMACH, GUT, LIVER, AND PANCREAS
Gastroparesis

Gastroparesis is a condition that occurs when nerves that help move food from the stomach through the intestine become damaged, typically after years of poorly controlled diabetes. This can lead to the bloating and discomfort that some people with diabetes experience on a regular basis after meals.

▶ WHAT YOU NEED TO KNOW

Gastroparesis results from damage to the nerves supplying the stomach, causing food to leave the stomach more slowly and erratically. This can lead to abdominal discomfort, which occurs because of a buildup of undigested food in the gut. Gastroparesis is important to diagnose because the delay in digestion can lead to erratic blood glucose levels that are difficult to manage.

Who Is at Risk?
People with a history of poorly controlled diabetes, usually those with other

complications of diabetes, such as eye disease, nerve damage (also known as neuropathy), and kidney disease, are most susceptible to this condition.

What Are the Symptoms?

The most common symptoms are

- feeling full quickly even after a light meal;
- abdominal pain or general discomfort;
- cramping after a meal;
- bloating after a meal; and
- nausea and vomiting, occasionally of undigested food long after a meal.

How Is It Diagnosed?

Some people have minor symptoms but perform poorly on diagnostic tests, while others report severe symptoms but have only a minor delay in digestion. This difference in symptoms and test results makes gastroparesis a difficult condition to diagnose.

To begin, the health care provider might order a nuclear medicine test that can be performed in an outpatient radiology department. People are asked to eat a meal—a plate of scrambled eggs, for example—that contains a radioactive tracer. The radiologist will take a series of images to monitor the tracer as it moves through the digestive tract. The slow movement of food out of the stomach and into the gut can indicate gastroparesis. Similarly, the health care provider might order a procedure called an *endoscopy* to determine if a significant amount of food remains in the stomach several hours after a meal. The endoscopy test involves the person being sedated and having a camera placed down the esophagus (food pipe). The camera goes into the stomach to take pictures. An endoscopy can also exclude the possibility of a mechanical blockage, which produces symptoms similar to gastroparesis but requires different treatment.

What Are the Treatment Options?

Gastroparesis can be a difficult condition to treat, as the few therapies that exist have some side effects.

The first therapy is typically changing the diet. People will usually meet with a dietitian to develop a plan that includes small, frequent meals low in fiber and fat. Nutritional supplements are sometimes recommended.

Once the diet is modified and glucose control is optimized, certain medications may further alleviate symptoms. In the United States, gastroparesis is most commonly treated with metoclopramide (brand name Reglan), a medication that acts both on the stomach and the brain to increase the movement of food through the gut. High doses can cause drowsiness, and long-term treatment can cause a serious and sometimes irreversible condition called *tardive dyskinesia*, which leads to repetitive, jerky movements in the face, tongue, and neck (let your provider know immediately if that occurs). Low-dose erythromycin, an antibiotic with additional effects that speed up stomach emptying, is sometimes prescribed, though it becomes gradually less effective the longer it is used. Domperidone is a medication that acts on the nerves of the stomach to speed up food leaving the stomach. It is prescribed in Canada and Europe but has not yet been approved by the Food and Drug Administration (FDA) for use in the United States.

If dietary changes and medications are not successful, the health care provider might recommend an implanted device called a *gastric pacemaker* that increases muscle contractions to help move food along in the gastrointestinal tract.

WHAT DOES IT ALL MEAN?

- Gastroparesis is a condition that occurs from damage to the nerves supplying the stomach, causing bloating, nausea, and possibly vomiting after most meals.
- Those with poorly managed diabetes over a long period of time are at greatest risk of developing gastroparesis.
- A number of treatment options exist, including dietary changes, improved glucose control, medications, or an implantable nerve stimulator to speed up stomach emptying.
- Some medications for diabetes, such as GLP-1 agonists, may slow emptying of the stomach and should not be used in people with gastroparesis.

Celiac Disease and Type 1 Diabetes

While perusing the grocery store, have you ever noticed foods labeled "gluten free" and wondered what they're for?

These foods are made for people who have a sensitivity to gluten, a condition called *celiac disease*. When people eat gluten, their immune system mistakenly attacks their own intestines because of the presence of autoantibodies.

Celiac disease is rare in the general population, but it's much more common in people who have another autoimmune disease: type 1 diabetes.

What Is Gluten?

Gluten—from a Latin word meaning "glue"—is found in wheat and many other cereal grains. It's what makes dough stretchy and fresh loaves of bread chewy. Gluten is found in almost all types of foods—even in the barley used to make beer.

Chances are, there's a gluten-free option for any food you're craving. Gluten-free breads, for example, are often made from rice flour instead of wheat.

What Are the Symptoms of Celiac Disease?

When people with celiac disease eat gluten, they develop a number of these uncomfortable gastrointestinal symptoms:

- ✓ Diarrhea
- ✓ Abdominal pain and bloating
- ✓ Difficulty gaining or keeping on weight
- ✓ Feeling tired
- ✓ Deficiencies in vitamin D, iron, and other nutrients
- ✓ Weak bones, or *osteoporosis*

How Is Celiac Disease Detected?

People are almost always diagnosed with type 1 diabetes before learning that they have celiac disease, but sometimes it happens the other way around.

If you have symptoms of celiac disease, your health care provider might order a blood test to determine if you're sensitive to gluten. If you have celiac disease, the blood test will reveal that your body produces certain proteins, called *auto-antibodies*, that specifically attack the tissues in your small intestines.

If these antibodies are found, your provider might recommend an endoscopy. After you're sedated, the physician will slide a tiny camera down your throat and into your intestines. This allows the provider to check for damage to your intestinal tissues that might have been caused by exposure to gluten and take a tissue biopsy.

What Treatments Are Available?

If you have celiac disease, your provider will recommend switching to a gluten-free diet. Because gluten is found in so many types of foods, it's extremely helpful to meet with a dietitian who can teach you about gluten-free alternatives and help you craft an enticing meal plan.

A few decades ago, people with celiac disease had few options when it came to dining out. But thanks to an increased awareness of this condition, gluten-free foods are now available at many mainstream grocery stores and restaurants. If you have both type 1 diabetes and celiac disease, your dietitian can develop a meal plan to help manage both conditions.

The best news of all? Your symptoms should completely disappear after a few weeks on a gluten-free diet.

WHAT DOES IT ALL MEAN?

Celiac disease is an autoimmune disorder that results in multiple uncomfortable gastrointestinal symptoms. This occurs due to a sensitivity to gluten, which is found in many foods, particularly wheat and grains. The condition is rare in the general population but occurs at a much higher frequency in people with type 1 diabetes. Meeting with a dietitian and eating a gluten-free diet is the best way to manage celiac disease, but more complex dietary adjustments may be required in the presence of type 1 diabetes.

Nonalcoholic Fatty Liver Disease

Fatty liver disease occurs when unhealthy amounts of fat accumulate in the liver. Most people associate this condition with a long history of alcohol abuse. But liver disease can also occur in people who do not drink alcohol in excess. This is known as *nonalcoholic fatty liver disease* (NAFLD) or sometimes *nonalcoholic steatohepatitis* (NASH).

People diagnosed with nonalcoholic fatty liver disease are usually obese and accumulate fat in their livers. It is common in people with type 2 diabetes and can occur in men who consume fewer than two alcoholic drinks daily or women who consume less than one alcoholic drink daily.

▶ WHAT YOU NEED TO KNOW

Nonalcoholic fatty liver disease often affects people who are overweight. But it's much more common among people with elevated blood glucose levels, thereby also affecting many people with type 2 diabetes.

Not only are people with type 2 diabetes more likely than others to develop nonalcoholic fatty liver disease, they're also more likely to develop a more aggressive form of this liver disease—NASH. In general, the following factors increase a person's risk of severe liver disease:

- Older age (older than 50 years)
- Extreme obesity
- High blood pressure

- Type 2 diabetes
- Abnormal liver tests on routine blood testing

How Is Nonalcoholic Fatty Liver Disease Detected?

Without routine blood tests, liver disease might go unnoticed until it causes serious illness. Some people might feel unusually tired, but many people have no noticeable symptoms early in the disease. If liver disease progresses to advanced stages, people may have loss of appetite, fatigue, yellowing of the skin, darkening of urine, and abdominal swelling.

In many cases, health care providers become suspicious when routine blood tests reveal abnormal liver function. If this happens, your provider may explore the various reasons for this test result, such as viral hepatitis, alcohol use, or other conditions that affect the liver. Your health care provider may also ask how many alcoholic drinks you consume every day. If it seems likely that you have liver disease, your provider may obtain MRI, CT, or ultrasound images of your liver to look at the fat content.

Indirectly measuring the fat content of the liver with imaging studies can give providers some helpful clues, but a biopsy may be needed to determine how well the liver is working. The biopsy results can indicate whether a person has liver disease and how severe it is.

How Is This Disease Treated?

Healthy lifestyle changes are the cornerstones of treatment for this condition:

- Lose weight. A weight loss of just 5% to 7% of your overall body weight can improve health by reversing the accumulation of fat in the liver.
- Exercise. Even if you don't lose weight, regular exercise can still improve the health of patients with fatty liver disease.
- Stop drinking. Most providers agree that men who drink fewer than two drinks a day and women who drink less than one drink a day are less likely to develop severe liver disease leading to cirrhosis. However, everyone responds to alcohol differently, and if even modest alcohol consumption is a suspected cause of the fat accumulation in your liver, your provider will probably recommend refraining from alcohol.
- Watch your blood glucose. Work with your provider to reduce your A1C level to 7% (53 mmol/mol) or less.

If these changes aren't enough to improve your liver function, your doctor might recommend medication. Drugs such as pioglitazone (see "Thiazolidine-diones" on page 242) and GLP-1 agonists (see "Incretin Mimetics [GLP-1 Agonists]" on page 233) have been used to treat nonalcoholic fatty liver disease, though they have not yet been FDA approved for this purpose.

These medications also help blood glucose management in people with type 2 diabetes. Ask your provider what would work best for you.

WHAT DOES IT ALL MEAN?

Nonalcoholic fatty liver disease is a common condition in people who are obese and have diabetes. In some cases, nonalcoholic fatty liver disease can progress to serious liver disease with liver failure. Basic treatments such as weight loss, exercise, and good management of diabetes can be effective.

Testing for Liver Disease

The liver is a vital organ that helps the body break down drugs and toxins. It also plays key roles in digestion, clotting, blood glucose management, and the production of many proteins. However, this organ is highly vulnerable to damage in people with diabetes.

▶ WHAT YOU NEED TO KNOW

Nonalcoholic fatty liver disease, a condition that occurs when unhealthy amounts of fat accumulate in the liver, is common in people with type 2 diabetes. This condition can worsen and even lead to liver failure (cirrhosis), so careful monitoring by health care providers is required. Liver disease is most common in people with diabetes who are overweight or drink alcohol.

Your provider may recommend routine blood tests to detect the earliest signs of liver damage before it causes serious problems.

Symptoms of Liver Disease
People with liver disease can have the following symptoms:
- Yellowish (also called *jaundiced*) skin and yellowing of the whites of the eyes
- Dark urine
- Very light or dark-colored stools
- A swollen or painful abdomen
- Loss of appetite
- Tiredness or fatigue
- Nausea or vomiting
- Recent unexplained weight changes

- Itchy skin
- Swollen legs or ankles

Understanding Your Test Results

Medical care providers watch for signs of liver disease by performing blood tests that monitor the activity of key enzymes in the liver. These enzymes aren't specific to nonalcoholic fatty liver disease though, so the tests sometimes uncover signs of other conditions, such as hepatitis C.

By collecting information on several liver enzymes, providers can piece together an overall picture of the liver's health.

- **Alanine Aminotransferase (ALT)** This enzyme is abundant in the liver. When both ALT and AST levels are elevated, the doctor may recommend further testing to narrow down the cause of liver damage.
- **Aspartate Aminotransferase (AST)** This enzyme is not only found in the liver, it's also present in the heart and other muscles.
- **Alkaline Phosphatase (ALP)** This enzyme is found throughout the body, including the liver. Elevated levels of both ALP and gamma-glutamyl transpeptidase (GGT; see the next bullet point) could reveal a number of possible conditions ranging from temporary problems in liver function to serious conditions such as cirrhosis. An elevation in ALP alone can be a sign of blockage of the ducts draining the liver. An elevation of ALP alone can also signal a separate condition, such as pregnancy, bone disease, or heart disease.
- **Gamma–glutamyl Transpeptidase (GGT)** This enzyme is found in the liver, kidney, pancreas, and intestine. Heavy alcohol use sometimes causes elevated GGT levels. When this test and the ALP are both high, it indicates a likely problem in the liver.

WHAT DOES IT ALL MEAN?

People with diabetes can develop fatty accumulations in the liver (nonalcoholic fatty liver disease) and other liver conditions. Problems in the liver are usually first detected by finding higher-than-normal levels of liver enzymes in the blood. Regularly screening liver enzymes can detect early signs of liver disease so that treatments can be started early to prevent the condition from worsening.

Pancreatitis

People with type 2 diabetes are much more likely than others to experience a sudden flare of inflammation of the pancreas, or *pancreatitis*, which may also be accompanied by high blood glucose levels. Conversely, in those without diabetes, repeated episodes of pancreatitis can cause chronic pain and inflammation of the pancreas and eventually lead to the destruction of pancreatic tissue with subsequent prediabetes or diabetes.

▶ WHAT YOU NEED TO KNOW

Of all the organs in the body, the pancreas is by far the most important when it comes to maintaining healthy blood glucose levels. When the pancreas is not working properly—because of inflammation, tissue destruction, surgical removal, or injury—blood glucose can become difficult to control.

The pancreas releases two important hormones that help keep blood glucose levels in a normal range: insulin and glucagon. Other enzymes are also produced that affect digestion.

Inflammation of the pancreas can result from alcohol consumption, gallstones, extremely high triglycerides, certain medications, and traumatic injury. This leads to pancreatitis.

What Are the Symptoms of Pancreatitis?
The symptoms of acute pancreatitis include
- pain in the upper abdomen that may feel worse after eating,
- nausea or vomiting,
- fever, and
- fast heart rate.

The symptoms of chronic pancreatitis include
- pain in the upper abdomen that may feel worse after eating,
- nausea or vomiting,
- weight loss,
- oily or fatty stools, and
- diarrhea.

How Is Pancreatitis Detected?
If you experience the symptoms listed and your provider suspects that you have pancreatitis, you may be sent for a blood test to measure the levels of two digestive enzymes—amylase and lipase—produced by the pancreas. In some cases, pancreatitis can be so severe that part of the pancreas becomes permanently damaged, which can lead to prediabetes or diabetes. If your enzyme lev-

els are high and your symptoms are severe, you will likely be sent for an imaging study, such as a CT scan or endoscopic ultrasound, so the provider can look at an image of your pancreas and determine if there is any damage.

Are There Treatments for Pancreatitis?

Yes. Most people are admitted to the hospital, where they receive intravenous fluids to rehydrate and replete their electrolytes and medications to manage their pain. To rest the gut, people are not allowed to eat until they recover.

In people with chronic pancreatitis, oral replacement of pancreatic enzymes is usually needed. Other vitamins (such as vitamin D) may also not be absorbed as well and require supplementation.

WHAT DOES IT ALL MEAN?

A healthy pancreas makes insulin and glucagon, which are used to maintain normal blood glucose values, in addition to digestive enzymes. Inflammation of the pancreas, known as pancreatitis, can result in abdominal pain and sometimes lead to high blood glucose levels in people without diabetes. Pancreatitis can result from alcohol, gallstones, or other causes. Repeated episodes of pancreatitis can result in chronic pancreatitis and diabetes. People with diabetes are much more likely to have episodes of pancreatitis and should be monitored closely. Pancreatitis may also be a potential warning when taking certain types of diabetes medications such as GLP-1 agonists and DPP-IV inhibitors.

THE KIDNEYS

Diabetic Kidney Disease

Up to half of people with diabetes will develop diabetic kidney disease at some point in their lives. Also known as *diabetic nephropathy*, kidney disease is most common among persons with diabetes who have had poorly controlled blood glucose levels for many years. High blood pressure also increases the chances of developing kidney disease.

▶ WHAT YOU NEED TO KNOW

The kidneys are two bean-shaped organs located in the back of the abdomen, just below the ribs. They filter and remove waste from the blood through the urine, as well as regulate the amount of fluid and salts in the body. Consequently, the kidneys are also important in controlling blood pressure.

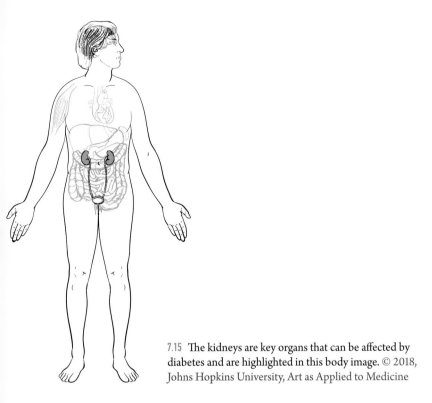

7.15 The kidneys are key organs that can be affected by diabetes and are highlighted in this body image. © 2018, Johns Hopkins University, Art as Applied to Medicine

Uncontrolled high blood glucose levels can damage tiny blood vessels in the kidneys, reducing their ability to filter the blood. As a result, a small type of protein called *albumin* spills into the urine instead of staying in the bloodstream, leading to increased urinary albumin excretion. A small amount of this protein in the urine is called *microalbuminuria*; as kidney disease progresses, more protein is found in the urine, a condition called *macroalbuminuria* or *proteinuria*. The glomerular filtration rate (GFR) is determined from blood tests, age, sex, and race and represents how effectively your kidneys filter toxins from your blood. Kidney disease is present if there is 1) elevated protein in the urine (greater than or equal to 30 milligrams [mg] albumin per gram [g] creatinine), and/or 2) a reduced GFR level.

The staging of chronic kidney disease is based on the GFR level as described in table 7.2.

Symptoms are rare during the earliest stages of kidney disease, but you might notice your blood pressure rise. If blood tests reveal a moderate decrease in your GFR or moderate levels of protein in your urine, you may still be able to slow

Table 7.2. The staging of chronic kidney disease

STAGE OF KIDNEY DISEASE	GFR* (ML/MIN/1.73M^2)	CONDITION OF THE KIDNEYS
1	90 or higher**	The kidneys function normally but are at risk for kidney disease
2	60–89**	Mild decline in kidney function
3	30–59	Moderate decline in kidney function
4	15–29	Severe decline in kidney function
5	14 or lower	Kidney failure (end-stage kidney disease)

*GFR = glomerular filtration rate.
**With evidence of kidney damage such as albuminuria.

the development of kidney disease by improving your blood glucose levels and blood pressure. Persons with kidney disease often develop high blood pressure (if they didn't have it already) and may need to be on more blood pressure medications than before.

As kidney disease progresses, your kidneys will continue to become less effective. Symptoms might include fatigue, poor appetite, and nausea. You will be tested for anemia (see "Anemia" on page 191) and may require treatment. You may need medications to keep phosphate levels from rising too high and to treat vitamin D deficiency. Mineral and bone disorders can occur as kidney disease progresses. Several changes to your diet may also be recommended. You may find that you actually need less insulin because this is cleared by the kidney, as well. Chronic kidney disease over time results in reduced kidney size and various types of damage to the kidneys, as depicted in figure 7.16.

When you reach the point where your kidneys can no longer function well enough on their own (called *end-stage kidney disease*), you may need to start dialysis. Because waste products from the blood are not as readily cleared from the body, fluid overload, or edema, becomes a problem and may result in swelling of the hands, arms, feet, ankles, and legs. You might also have difficulty breathing.

A hemodialysis machine or fluid exchange in the abdomen (*peritoneal dialysis*) can take over the kidneys' job of filtering toxins from the blood and removing excess fluid. A kidney transplant is also a treatment option for people with diabetes and end-stage kidney disease.

WHAT DOES IT ALL MEAN?

Persons with diabetes need to be regularly tested for kidney function and protein in the urine (microalbumin test)—usually at least once a year. Strategies to prevent kidney disease include managing blood glucose, blood pressure, and cholesterol levels and eating healthily, exercising regularly, and quitting smoking. Regular screening, early detection, and appropriate treatment of diabetic kidney disease can dramatically reduce any further decline in kidney function and delay or prevent the need for dialysis or a kidney transplant.

Testing for Kidney Function

Your kidneys play an important role in clearing waste products, fluids, and medications from your body. Diabetes is the most common cause of kidney disease in adults. Blood and urine tests are regularly used to monitor for signs of kidney disease.

▶ WHAT YOU NEED TO KNOW

Diabetes can take a toll on the kidneys, so don't be surprised if your provider monitors your kidneys on a regular basis. It's important to detect problems with these organs as early as possible to prevent kidney failure.

Many people experience the first signs of kidney damage about 5 or 10 years after receiving a diabetes diagnosis, especially if their diabetes has not been well managed.

Following your provider's recommended diet and exercise guidelines is always important, but it becomes even more critical once you reach this point. Well-managed blood glucose levels and blood pressure can slow further kidney damage but if not, kidney failure can occur in the years to come.

Testing for Early Detection of Kidney Disease

Your health care provider will collect blood and urine samples to measure the health of your kidneys. Your kidney function will be tested at least annually. Your provider may order these tests more often if you are taking medications that subject the kidneys to stress:

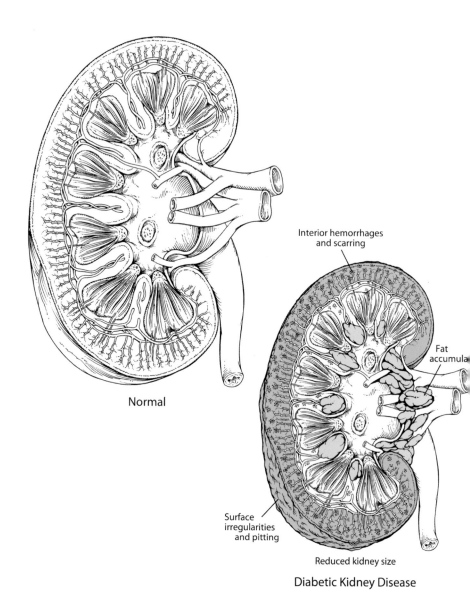

Interior hemorrhages
and scarring

Fat
accumula

Surface
irregularities
and pitting

Normal

Reduced kidney size

Diabetic Kidney Disease

7.16 Multiple changes can occur in the kidney with diabetic kidney disease, including scarring inside the kidney, changes to the surface of the kidney, reduced kidney size, and fat accumulation. These changes can result in decreased kidney function. © 2018, Johns Hopkins University, Art as Applied to Medicine

- The blood test for kidney function is the *serum creatinine level*. It is used along with age, sex, and race to calculate the GFR, which is a measure of how well the kidneys filter waste from the blood.
- As kidney disease progresses, the GFR declines. The results of the creatinine test are usually the opposite of the GFR. That is, when creatinine results are high, GFR results are low and vice versa.
- Your provider will also request a urine sample to test your *urine albumin to creatinine ratio* (see "Testing for Albuminuria" on page 156).
- Certain imaging tests—such as an ultrasound or CT scans—are used to detect blockages in the flow of urine in the kidney or bladder, blood flow problems to the kidney, or visible damage to these organs. If you have kidney disease and need an imaging test, your provider will likely advise you to have only CT scans without contrast or MRI without the contrast agent known as *gadolinium*. This will help prevent further kidney injury.
- Blood tests can also detect other problems that occur when kidney function declines, such as anemia (see "Anemia" on page 191) or high acid levels in the blood.

While most people with the earlier stages of kidney disease have no symptoms, the signs and symptoms of more severe kidney disease include frothy urine (like the bubbles in a soda), leg swelling, difficult-to-control high blood pressure, shortness of breath, loss of appetite, and nausea.

Interpreting the Results

Your medical care provider will rely on these test results to track how your kidneys are working and intervene if you show signs of kidney disease. Certain factors can influence these results, however, so any abnormal tests should be repeated. Depending on the severity of your kidney disease, your provider may refer you to a nephrologist for further care.

WHAT DOES IT ALL MEAN?

Kidney health is important to keep the overall body healthy. Kidney disease is common in people with diabetes. Blood and urine tests are available that can detect kidney disease and help guide treatments to improve or preserve kidney function. Regular testing of your kidneys can help detect kidney disease at its earliest stages.

Testing for Albuminuria

Albuminuria means the finding of an increased amount of albumin (a small protein) in the urine. Usually, little to no albumin is lost in the urine. It can be an early sign of kidney disease.

▶ WHAT YOU NEED TO KNOW

Detecting the Earliest Signs of Kidney Disease

Early signs of kidney disease can be detected with a simple urine microalbumin test. This test determines if the kidneys are leaking a protein called albumin, which signals that changes due to diabetes may be damaging the kidneys. Your health care provider will need to check this urine test at least twice to confirm the findings because a number of factors, such as exercise, fever, or elevated blood pressure, can cause short-term changes in urine albumin. An elevated level is considered a urine albumin-to-creatinine ratio greater than or equal to 30 mg/g creatinine (commonly called microalbuminuria) or greater than or equal to 300 mg/g creatinine (commonly called macroalbuminuria).

What Do the Results Mean?

If your urine test is persistently positive, you may be told you have albuminuria. This is a sign of chronic kidney disease. It is important to detect this because albuminuria raises a person's chances of developing end-stage kidney failure and heart disease in people with diabetes.

The good news is that albuminuria can be managed if detected early. Managing blood pressure is critically important. Your provider may recommend certain drugs, such as ACE inhibitors (see "Angiotensin-Converting Enzyme Inhibitors" on page 269) or ARBs (see "Angiotensin-Receptor Blockers" on page 272), to help protect your kidneys from further damage. If your glucose levels have been running high, better diabetes management will also be recommended to protect your kidneys.

How Often Should I Be Tested?

People with type 2 diabetes are screened for kidney disease with a urine microalbumin test when they're first diagnosed, then every year thereafter. People with type 1 diabetes usually start annual urine microalbumin screenings for kidney disease 5 years after they've been diagnosed and then yearly thereafter.

Starting and Managing Dialysis

Dialysis is a treatment in which waste products, as well as excess fluid, are removed from the blood artificially when your kidneys are no longer able to do so. More than half of people with end-stage kidney disease who need dialysis have diabetes.

▶ WHAT YOU NEED TO KNOW

Key Facts about Dialysis

1 Dialysis is a treatment for people with end-stage kidney disease. The dialysis machine removes harmful substances or toxins from their blood, a job normally performed by the kidneys.

2 People with end-stage kidney disease must remain on dialysis unless they receive a kidney transplant. People who have kidney transplants tend to live longer than those treated with dialysis. For that reason, providers strongly encourage people who are eligible for a transplant to have the surgery. People with end-stage kidney disease can also receive a transplant instead of going on dialysis.

3 About half of all people on dialysis have diabetes. People who have diabetic kidney disease tend to die sooner than those without diabetes. In fact, about half of the people on dialysis who die do so from heart disease or stroke.

4 People with diabetes tend to fare worse than other people on dialysis. For this reason, your nephrologist might recommend treating you with medications and changes to your diet until dialysis is thought to be absolutely necessary. Reasons for beginning dialysis include fluid overload or heart failure; a buildup of harmful substances in the blood that alters a person's mental state, known as *uremia*; or electrolyte imbalances (such as high potassium or high acid levels) that result when the kidneys are unable to do their job. These problems typically arise after a person's GFR (see "Testing for Kidney Function" on page 153) falls to less than 10 ml/min/1.73 m^2.

5   People with diabetes who are on dialysis should take insulin rather than other diabetes medications. Common oral medications, such as some sulfonylureas, are cleared from the body by the kidneys and therefore may have a prolonged effect in a patient with reduced kidney function. This may lead to dangerously low blood glucose levels. Metformin can lead to a buildup of acid in the blood, a condition known as *lactic acidosis*, when the kidneys are not working well. Insulin is the best option for treating diabetes for people who are on dialysis.

What Are the Types of Dialysis?

Hemodialysis is performed over the course of a few hours in a dialysis center or at home. The patient's blood is cycled out of the body, filtered through a machine, and cycled back into the body through a connection to the blood vessels. Access to the blood is created through minor surgery, usually on your arm, to make a connection between an artery and a vein called an *AV fistula*. It is important to plan ahead and have the fistula placed early so that it has time to mature before beginning hemodialysis. Another option is to place a soft tube that joins an artery and a vein in the arm, called an *AV graft*. In some people, a catheter may be placed in a large vein (such as the neck) for hemodialysis, but fistulas are usually the preferred choice. People treated with hemodialysis at a center generally complete three sessions per week. Hemodialysis can also be done at home and involves shorter and more frequent treatments than hemodialysis at a center.

Peritoneal dialysis is performed at home, either multiple times during the day or overnight. Fluid is placed through a port, or opening, into the person's abdominal cavity. The fluid collects harmful substances or toxins from the patient's body and then is drained out. Being able to do this treatment at home is desirable to many people. This type of dialysis is not ideal for people who have trouble using their hands, who are morbidly obese, or who have very poorly managed diabetes.

WHAT DOES IT ALL MEAN?

- End-stage kidney disease is treated with dialysis or a kidney transplant.
- Diabetes is the leading cause of end-stage kidney disease requiring dialysis.
- Two forms of dialysis are available: hemodialysis and peritoneal dialysis.

Kidney Transplantation

Transplanting a kidney from a donor can cure chronic kidney disease. A transplanted kidney may be obtained from a deceased or a living donor. People have two kidneys but can survive with one healthy kidney. Diabetic kidney disease is the most common reason for kidney transplantation. The availability of donor organs for kidney transplant is a major limitation to this surgery, and there are national kidney transplant waiting lists (see www.unos.org).

▶ WHAT YOU NEED TO KNOW

Who Is Eligible for a Kidney Transplant?

A team of health care providers, including transplant specialists, will consider many factors before recommending an organ transplant for a person with chronic kidney disease:

- Only people with very low kidney function are considered for a transplant.
- People with heart disease may be eligible, but the provider may recommend further testing and treatment before the transplant.
- Transplants are not typically recommended for people with substance use disorders or others who lack much-needed social support during recovery.
- Obese people may have more complications from transplant surgery, and therefore a provider may recommend weight loss prior to a kidney transplant.
- People with certain underlying health conditions (such as severe lung disease or specific cancers) may not be eligible for a transplant.

What to Expect after a Kidney Transplant

Your team of transplant providers will follow your recovery closely during the weeks after surgery. They may test for complications such as infection or organ rejection. After a transplant, people must take antirejection medications to prevent the immune system from attacking the transplanted kidney. These drugs are usually taken for the rest of the person's life and may include tacrolimus (brand name Prograf) or cyclosporine (brand names Neoral or Gengraf), which can both exacerbate blood glucose levels in people with diabetes. Steroids, such as prednisone, may also be prescribed after kidney transplant and may worsen blood glucose control if appropriate adjustments are not made in diabetes medications. After discharge, the health care provider will recommend home monitoring of the person's blood glucose levels. Long-term monitoring of blood glucose, such as the A1C, may not be accurate until a few months after surgery.

WHAT DOES IT ALL MEAN?

Whether or not you have strong risk factors, your health care provider will probably measure your fasting blood glucose frequently during the first few months after surgery. However, if you develop increased thirst or excessive urination between these tests, be sure to notify your transplant team, as these symptoms are common when glucose levels run high and can be seen in new-onset diabetes after transplant.

THE BLADDER
Bladder Disorders in Diabetes

Many people with diabetes have trouble urinating or controlling their urine. These problems vary widely. Some people have trouble making it to the bathroom on time, while others accidentally leak urine when exercising, laughing, or sneezing. This is called *urinary incontinence*. People with diabetic nerve damage may not notice the urge to urinate until it's too late to reach a bathroom. If this happens to you, it's important to know that you're not alone—and treatments are available.

▶ WHAT YOU NEED TO KNOW

Tests to Diagnose Bladder Problems

Your provider may perform a series of tests to ensure that your bladder problems are due to diabetes rather than other common urinary issues, such as an enlarged prostate gland in men or a urinary tract infection in women.

You might also be asked a few questions about your bathroom habits, such as:
- How often do you urinate?
- Can you fully empty your bladder?
- What sensations do you feel when your bladder is full? Some people feel a sudden urgency to use the bathroom, while others barely feel the need to go.

Tips for Better Urine Control

Most people benefit from frequent trips to the bathroom so their bladders never overflow. Women may find it helpful to exercise the muscles that control the pelvic floor by repetitively tightening and releasing these muscles a few times a day. These are called *Kegel exercises.*

Studies suggest that weight loss and exercise are even more effective than drugs at improving bladder control, partly because a healthier lifestyle improves blood glucose management. Improved diabetes management reduces the risk of damage to nerves that supply the bladder. In most persons, when glucose levels rise above 180 mg/dL, glucose appears in the urine. This draws more water into

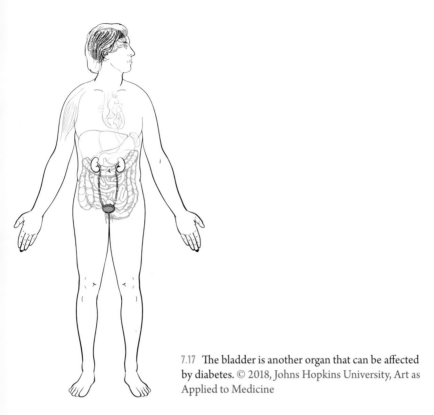

7.17 The bladder is another organ that can be affected by diabetes. © 2018, Johns Hopkins University, Art as Applied to Medicine

the urine and fills the bladder more rapidly, resulting in people with diabetes needing to urinate more. When high glucose levels develop in persons with diabetes who have bladder problems, bladder function often worsens. Healthy blood glucose levels therefore promote healthier bladder function.

But if these interventions aren't enough, your provider may prescribe medications, such as oxybutynin or bethanechol, that help to relax the bladder and prevent incontinence.

WHAT DOES IT ALL MEAN?

Bladder disorders are more common in persons with diabetes. These can lead to difficulty fully emptying the bladder and urinary incontinence. Your provider can help determine whether a condition other than diabetes may be causing your symptoms. More frequent trips to the bathroom, special exercises, weight loss, regular physical activity, better diabetes management, and certain medications can all reduce the symptoms of bladder disorders.

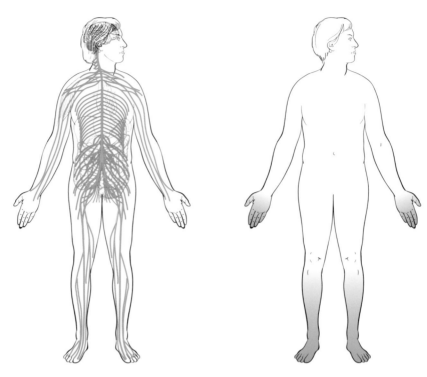

7.18 (*left*) The nerves in the body are key organs that diabetes can affect.
© 2018, Johns Hopkins University, Art as Applied to Medicine

7.19 (*right*) The common "stocking-glove" location of numbness or pain in persons with neuropathy. © 2018, Johns Hopkins University, Art as Applied to Medicine

THE NERVES
Peripheral Neuropathy

Some people with diabetes have trouble with the feeling in their feet and hands and experience strange burning or tingling sensations in their feet and hands. This results from damage to the long nerves that extend from the spinal cord to various parts of the body. Damage to these long nerves, known as *peripheral neuropathy*, is the most commonly reported type of nerve damage among persons with diabetes (figure 7.19).

▶ WHAT YOU NEED TO KNOW

The longest nerves in the human body extend all the way from the brain to the feet. Peripheral neuropathy from diabetes almost always affects the long nerves first, starting in both feet and working gradually up the legs. Left untreated, nerve damage can also affect other parts of the body, including the hands. Symptoms can include numbness, burning, shooting pains, or a "pins and needles" feeling, usually in both feet. Sometimes people will describe being extremely sensitive to light touch, such as when their feet feel the bedsheets at night, called *allodynia*.

Key Facts about Peripheral Neuropathy

1 It's very common. About one-quarter of all persons with diabetes have symptoms, but additional nerve testing would probably reveal peripheral neuropathy in more than half of all persons with diabetes who may not have symptoms.

2 It's preventable. People are more likely to develop nerve damage if they've had diabetes for many years; smoke; or have poorly controlled blood glucose, high blood pressure, or high cholesterol.

3 Sometimes it's diagnosed with prediabetes. Though not very common, some patients complain of numbness in their feet—a symptom of peripheral neuropathy—before diabetes has developed, when glucose levels are high but not yet in the diabetic range.

4 It dramatically increases the chance of foot ulcers. People who have trouble with the feeling in their feet are less likely to notice injuries, calluses, or ulcers until a serious infection develops. This can lead to amputations. People with neuropathy should check their feet for signs of injury every day.

5 There are several ways to diagnose neuropathy. Simple office tests, including physical examination with tuning forks, pins, and monofilaments, assess whether a person can feel vibrations, proprioception (position sense), or sharp sensations in the feet. A more sophisticated test called a *nerve conduction study* measures how well the nerves transmit signals but is not generally required to diagnose diabetic neuropathy.

6 There are several medicines available to treat the pain (see "Treating Neuropathic Pain" on page 164). Talk to your health care provider if you are having painful symptoms suggestive of neuropathy.

WHAT DOES IT ALL MEAN?

Nerve damage can be prevented. Healthy lifestyle changes and careful management of blood glucose, blood pressure, and cholesterol levels can prevent and slow the progression of nerve damage and may improve symptoms. Awareness of the potential for nerve damage in diabetes and frequent inspections of the feet can prevent future infections, foot ulcers, and amputations.

Treating Neuropathic Pain

Nerve pain is common among people with diabetes. Years of poorly controlled blood glucose can gradually damage the nerves that transmit information from various parts of the body to the brain (see "Peripheral Neuropathy" on page 162). Sometimes medications are needed to treat the symptoms of neuropathic pain.

▶ WHAT YOU NEED TO KNOW

Damaged nerves can cause debilitating pain, particularly in the hands or feet. This condition is known as diabetic peripheral neuropathy (Figure 7.20). Numbness in the feet can prevent someone from feeling sores or blisters that develop. Sores on the feet can become infected. An untreated and severe foot infection may lead to an amputation.

Finding Relief

Two drugs—pregabalin (brand name Lyrica) and duloxetine (brand name Cymbalta)—are approved by the FDA to treat diabetic nerve pain.

Providers sometimes treat nerve pain with drugs that have been FDA approved for other conditions. The epilepsy drug gabapentin (brand name Neurontin), for example, is commonly used in this way. Antidepressants or antiseizure medications are sometimes used as well.

Providers normally treat nerve pain with the lowest possible amount of medication to avoid the side effects that often accompany higher doses. Sometimes these medications can take a few weeks to have an effect. Sedation or feeling drowsy can be a common side effect for some of these medications.

Alternative Treatments

Unfortunately, none of these drugs reverse nerve damage or completely eliminate symptoms. Some patients find relief in other types of treatment. Talk to your provider before considering these treatments:

- Nutritional supplements, such as Metanx or alpha-lipoic acid
- Topical creams or patches containing lidocaine or capsaicin (the spicy chemical in chili peppers)
- Devices that provide spinal or transcutaneous electrical nerve stimulation

Not all people with diabetic neuropathy need medications to treat their pain. However, if the symptoms become worse, they can be treated with different types of medications. Sometimes a referral to a nerve specialist (*neurologist*) is needed. None of the medications currently available to treat nerve pain can reverse nerve damage, although nerve pain often gets better over time (because nerve pain becomes numbness).

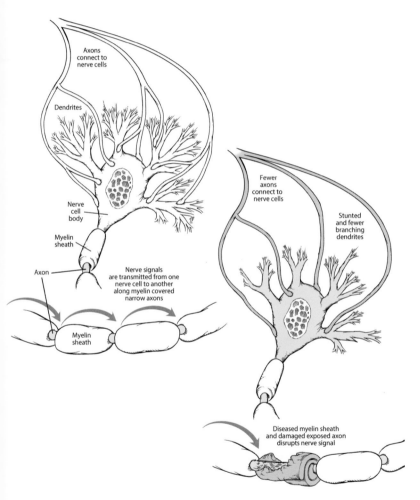

7.20 The anatomy of normal nerves and changes that can occur in persons with diabetic neuropathy, including fewer dendrites connecting nerve cells, stunted or shortened dendrites, and a diseased myelin sheath that disrupts nerve signaling. © 2018, Johns Hopkins University, Art as Applied to Medicine

Autonomic Neuropathy

Autonomic neuropathy occurs when special types of nerves that serve the gastrointestinal tract, heart, bladder, penis, and other organs of the body are damaged. This leads to certain symptoms when the organs the nerves supply don't function properly.

▶ WHAT YOU NEED TO KNOW

Think of all the processes that unfold naturally in your body: your regular heartbeat, bowel movements, and sexual arousal. These and other processes are controlled by nerves in the autonomic nervous system. This system functions like clockwork, controlling the heart and other bodily functions without you needing to think about them.

Damage to these nerves, a condition called autonomic neuropathy, is common in people with diabetes and can appear many years or decades after a diabetes diagnosis, particularly when diabetes is not well managed. Peripheral neuropathy is also usually present.

Interrupting the body's clockwork functions can cause major health problems and even death, so health care providers take this condition very seriously.

Nerve Damage and the Gastrointestinal Tract

This is the most common type of autonomic nerve damage in people with diabetes. It's often detected when people have the following symptoms:

- Heartburn
- Difficulty swallowing solid foods
- Feeling full after eating a small portion
- Loss of appetite
- Nausea or vomiting
- Stomachache or bloating
- Severe diarrhea that lasts hours or days, sometimes mingled with bouts of constipation

These symptoms can also occur with other gastrointestinal ailments, so your health care provider might recommend further testing to pin down the underlying cause. Tests that track movement through your gut, called *esophageal scintigraphy* and *gastric emptying studies*, are often suggested.

Sometimes these tests detect the slow passage of food from the stomach to the intestines, which make it difficult to keep blood glucose well managed (see "Gastroparesis" on page 141).

Your health care provider might refer you to a specialist, known as a *gastro-*

enterologist, for a treatment plan tailored to your individual needs. Some people benefit from

- eating four to six smaller meals per day instead of three large meals;
- a low-fat diet;
- eating less fiber during bouts of diarrhea;
- gluten-free or dairy-free diets;
- certain antibiotics and prescription medicines, such as erythromycin or metoclopramide, that promote the movement of food through the gut; or
- a stomach pacemaker (also known as a gastric pacer).

Nerve Damage and the Heart

Nerve damage affecting the heart and blood vessels can raise the risk of death dramatically, so it is important to detect this condition as early as possible.

Health care providers may consider heart-related nerve damage if certain symptoms develop, including

- dizziness or weakness when standing,
- fatigue, especially during exercise, or
- an unusually fast heartbeat during times of rest.

As nerve damage worsens, the heart loses its ability to pump faster during exercise and slower at rest. Some people also experience a dangerous drop in blood pressure when they stand up (*orthostatic hypotension*).

If your health care provider suspects you have heart-related nerve damage, he or she might recommend further testing or treatment as follows:

- Tilt-table testing to measure the heart's response to changes in position
- Heart-rate variability testing
- Medications and lifestyle changes to improve blood glucose management
- A high-salt diet, salt tablets, or medications to support blood pressure, such as fludrocortisone or midodrine, in people with orthostatic hypotension

Nerve Damage and Other Conditions

Nerve damage can affect other body functions, including urination and sexual arousal, or interfere with the ability to sweat:

- Bladder or urination problems, such as a weak stream, a slow start, dribbling, and trouble emptying the bladder can result from autonomic nerve damage. In some cases, health care providers recommend pressing on the bladder to strengthen the flow of urine. Left untreated, these problems increase the risk of a bladder infection, also known as a *urinary tract infection* (see "Bladder Disorders in Diabetes" on page 160). If you have more than two bladder infections in a year, your health care provider might perform additional tests for nerve damage.

- Erectile dysfunction in men often stems from a number of diabetes-related problems, including nerve damage and decreased blood flow to the genital area. It's important to alert your health care provider if you have trouble getting or keeping an erection, as this can signal a serious health problem. In many cases, erectile dysfunction (and the underlying problem) can be treated with medications (see "Erectile Dysfunction" on page 200).

- Sweat keeps your body cool during exercise and in warm weather. But diabetic nerve damage can interrupt this process, reducing sweat on the hands and feet and sometimes causing too much sweat on the trunk. This can result in a very low heat tolerance and easily becoming uncomfortable. Treatments range from Botox injections to prescription medications. Alert your health care provider if your feet sweat less than usual. Dry feet can develop sores called *ulcers* that may progress into more serious conditions.

WHAT DOES IT ALL MEAN?

Autonomic neuropathy refers to the abnormal function of the nerves supplying the stomach and intestines, heart, bladder, penis, and other body organs. Making your medical provider aware of any symptoms can speed the diagnosis of autonomic nerve damage and ensure the proper treatment is provided. This can help these organs function more normally or lessen aggravating symptoms.

THE FEET
Amputation

Amputation refers to the surgical removal of all or part of a limb, such as the leg, foot, toe, arm, hand, or finger. Though traumatic events, such as car accidents and military casualties, are among the most well-known reasons for losing a limb, the vast majority of toe, foot, and leg amputations actually occur in people with diabetes.

▶ WHAT YOU NEED TO KNOW

The thought of losing a foot or leg can seem devastating, but for patients with advanced complications from diabetes or life-threatening infections, it may be necessary.

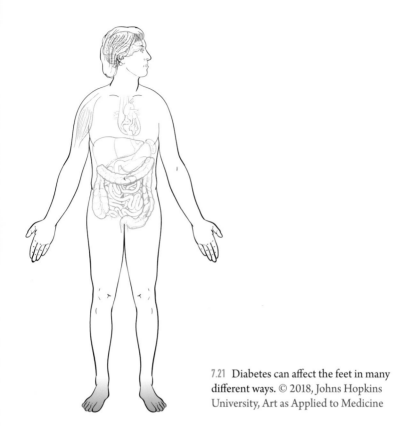

7.21 Diabetes can affect the feet in many different ways. © 2018, Johns Hopkins University, Art as Applied to Medicine

Who Is at Risk?

People who have had poorly controlled diabetes for many years are at highest risk for amputation, as well as people who

- ✓ are older than 65 years,
- ✓ smoke cigarettes,
- ✓ have had previous foot ulcers or amputations,
- ✓ have reduced blood circulation in their arteries (PAD),
- ✓ have peripheral neuropathy with a loss of feeling in the feet and hands,
- ✓ have foot deformities or infected ulcers on their feet,
- ✓ have kidney disease,
- ✓ have hair loss or shiny skin on the top of the foot or shin, and
- ✓ have thickened toenails.

My Risk of Amputation Is High. Now What?

Your health care provider will monitor you closely for signs of poor blood circulation to the legs. Often the provider might suggest a blood pressure test known as an *ankle brachial index* (ABI). Though the name sounds complex, the ABI is a simple method of diagnosing vascular insufficiency in the lower limbs:

- A Doppler ultrasonic probe is used to measure the blood pressure in your ankles and your arms.
- If the numbers are similar, you have adequate blood flow to your feet and legs and are at lower risk of having an amputation.
- If the blood pressure is lower in your ankle than your arm, your doctor will work with you to aggressively prevent foot ulcers, which are a leading cause of foot amputation.

Is an Amputation Really Necessary? How Can You Be Sure?

The decision to remove a limb is not an easy one. Before making this decision, your provider will order a number of medical tests to determine whether the toe, foot, or leg can be saved with other treatments. In addition to comparing blood pressure measurements in your ankle and arm, the provider may also evaluate the blood vessels in your feet and legs using x-rays, Doppler ultrasound, CT angiography (CTA), or magnetic resonance angiography (MRA). These procedures can reveal whether you have a blockage of blood flow to your legs and feet. Vascular surgery may be considered to improve blood flow.

If blood flow is poor and not surgically correctable, the size and depth of the wound are extensive, or the infection is severe, a minor or major amputation may be the best option. However, amputations are preventable with proper foot care and diabetes management and should really never reach this point. Amputation changes a person's ability to engage in weight-bearing activity and is the greatest risk factor for having another amputation.

How Much of My Foot or Leg Will Be Removed?

Every person is different but in general, your surgeon will try to remove the smallest possible area of dead tissue—a toe, for example—while allowing the surrounding tissue in your foot to heal. The goals of minor amputation are: 1) to remove unhealthy tissue, 2) to provide a foot that has the best chance to heal, 3) to provide a functional and cosmetically acceptable partial foot, and 4) to prevent major amputation of the leg.

Even if the surgeon finds it necessary to amputate a larger area, such as an entire foot or leg, he or she will work hard to leave a healthy stump or residual limb so the person with diabetes will have the best possible chance of walking independently, whether or not a prosthetic limb is needed. The goals of major amputation of the leg are: 1) to remove unhealthy tissue, 2) to provide a stump that has the best chance to heal, and 3) to provide a stump with the best chance of long-term function.

- Having poorly controlled diabetes increases the risk of developing foot ulcers and foot infections. This is made worse by impaired blood flow to the feet and diabetic nerve disease. Smoking increases the chances of developing peripheral arterial disease, impairs wound healing, and increases the risk of amputation.
- Sometimes foot or leg infections become so severe that an amputation is the best method to save the limb.
- Close follow-up is needed, with a focus on preventing amputation in the remaining limb.
- All people with diabetes should have their feet evaluated at least yearly.
- Seeing a foot care specialist (*podiatrist*) is recommended for regular preventive foot care and for the management of foot ulcers and infections.

Foot Ulcers

A diabetic foot ulcer (DFU) is a nonhealing or poorly healing wound below the ankle. It can occur when nerves in the feet are damaged from diabetes, resulting in the loss of protective sensation. Tight-fitting shoes can cause irritation of the skin by rubbing on a part of the foot that has become numb. Foot deformities result in elevated pressure on different parts of the foot. Open sores that go unnoticed can then progress to infections. PAD can further result in inadequate blood flow in the feet and poor healing of wounds. DFUs are often painless and are the leading cause of foot amputations.

▶ WHAT YOU NEED TO KNOW

Approximately 15% to 25% of persons with diabetes in the United States will develop a foot ulcer at some point in their lives. DFUs are the most common risk factor for amputation. DFUs often start out small but can quickly become infected. It may take several weeks or months for foot ulcers to heal. Your health care provider will need to probe the wound's depth to determine if the ulcer extends to the bone. He or she will remove unhealthy tissue using sterile instruments. A specialized wound dressing may be needed to promote healing, and antibiotics may be required to treat infection. It is essential to eliminate activities that lead to weight-bearing on the affected foot and to relieve pressure on the wound to allow it to heal. A cast or boot, a pair of crutches, or a wheelchair may be needed to take pressure off the ulcer while it heals.

Why Are Shoes So Important?
Properly fitting shoes are the number one way to prevent foot ulcers:
- Avoid flip-flops, high heels, stiff dress shoes, and open-toed shoes.
- Choose shoes that have plenty of toe room, a smooth inner lining, and a sole thick enough to prevent a puncture wound if you step on a tack or a nail.
- Always wear socks to absorb perspiration and to prevent skin irritation and blisters.
- Wear shoes that you can adjust easily, such as those with laces or Velcro.
- If your foot is deformed by bunions or hammertoes and "off the shelf" shoes don't fit, you may require special extra-depth shoes with molded insoles. These are often covered by insurance if you have neuropathy or PAD, foot deformities, or a history of foot ulcers.

What Should I Watch For?
Take a moment each day to inspect your feet. Don't forget to look between your toes. If you cannot see your feet, ask a family member or caretaker to check them for you. Alternatively, you can place a small nonbreakable mirror on the floor and hover your foot over it to see the underside. If you notice a callus, blister, drainage on your sock with or without pus or odor or an area of redness, increased warmth, or swelling contact your health care provider.

Are You at Risk for a Foot Ulcer?
- Do you often walk barefoot? The habit of going barefoot increases the risk of developing a foot ulcer. Wearing shoes—both inside and outside the house—can help protect your feet from injury.
- Do your shoes fit well? Poorly fitting shoes are a leading cause of foot ulcers.
- Do you have a foot deformity? If so, you may have a higher-than-average risk of a foot ulcer.
- Have you had a foot ulcer or amputation before? This puts you at higher risk of having another. Check your feet daily.
- Can you feel your feet? Diabetes can cause nerve damage to your feet, making it difficult to feel minor injuries.

- Can you see your feet? People who are overweight or have diabetic eye disease should ask a family member or caretaker to help examine their feet every day.
- Do you smoke? Ask your health care provider for help to quit.

- Foot ulcers can be prevented by taking good care of your feet and inspecting them daily to detect and treat problems early. Persons with diabetes who have foot deformities (for example, bunions or hammertoes), loss of feeling in their feet and legs (neuropathy), or PAD are at higher risk.
- Properly fitting footwear is the key to preventing DFUs.
- Keeping your blood glucose levels well managed will help stop DFUs from developing.
- Recognizing foot ulcers and infections early and receiving professional treatment from a podiatrist can help with faster healing and better outcomes.
- Seeing a podiatrist is recommended for regular preventive foot care in many people with diabetes.

Wound Healing

Wound healing is the body's natural process of regenerating skin and repairing tissue damage. This process can be compromised in people with diabetes due to the following factors: poor circulation, nerve damage, repeated trauma, and high blood glucose levels (hyperglycemia). Impaired wound healing is associated with infections and is the most important cause of amputation.

▶ WHAT YOU NEED TO KNOW

Wound healing should be carefully monitored regardless of where an injury occurs, but special attention should be paid to the feet. People with diabetes, particularly those who are overweight or have foot deformities, PAD, or trouble feeling their feet, are prone to developing foot ulcers. Left untreated, these wounds can become so severely infected that one or more toes or the entire foot must be removed. In fact, the majority of amputations in people with diabetes are preceded by a foot ulcer that failed to heal.

There are several actions, in addition to good blood glucose management, that will promote healthy wound healing and prevent further complications:
- Hygiene is crucial; cleanse and dress the wound daily.

- Eat a healthy diet.
- Be aware of new wounds, calluses, or signs of infection; inspect your feet daily.
- Eliminate activities that lead to weight bearing to relieve pressure on the wound.
- Leave the cigarettes behind; smoking increases the risk of PAD, and nicotine reduces nutritional blood flow to the skin and impairs wound healing.

The longer a wound remains untreated, the less likely it is to heal. Therefore, a health care provider will usually inspect any new wound to determine if it is infected and whether hospitalization is needed. The following factors can hint at the wound's severity:

- Location of the wound
- Size and depth of the wound
- Tenderness
- Temperature of the surrounding skin
- Redness around the wound or red streaks coming from the site of injury
- Presence of inflammation, pus, or discharge

Severe wounds will be cleansed and dressed by a team of specialists who have been trained to perform wound debridement for the removal of unhealthy tissue. Antibiotics are prescribed only for infected wounds. If the wound is on the leg or foot, a special boot, crutches, or a scooter or wheelchair will be needed to relieve pressure while standing so that it can heal.

WHAT DOES IT ALL MEAN?

- Wound healing may be delayed in people with diabetes.
- Chronic wounds are more likely to become infected and may require hospitalization and surgery.
- Wounds that do not fully heal after ulceration of the skin are a major risk factor for amputation.
- Taking pressure off the wound is critical to healing.
- Ill-fitting footwear may lead to recurring ulcers. Specialized shoes and orthotics are available to prevent this problem.
- Seeing a podiatrist can be helpful for wound care management.

Charcot Joint Disease (Neuroarthropathy)

People with diabetes who have nerve damage in their feet are at increased risk for a condition known as *Charcot joint disease,* which results in the deformity and instability of the foot, ankle, or both. It occurs suddenly and unexpectedly, often following a minor injury to the foot. The condition can be painless and presents with rapidly progressing inflammation, including redness, swelling, warmth, joint dislocations, fractures, and foot deformities. Early recognition of this condition and timely treatment is important.

▶ WHAT YOU NEED TO KNOW

Charcot joint disease is often triggered by a foot or ankle injury that is so minor the person barely remembers it. But within days the joint becomes red, hot, swollen, bruised, fractured, or dislocated. Oddly, this can be painless.

When someone continues to walk on this deformed foot, it can develop ulcers that take a long time to heal. Some people with this deformity develop serious infections that require amputation.

How Will I Know If I Have This Condition?

Charcot neuroarthropathy generally affects people who have had diabetes for many years, who are overweight, and who have severe peripheral neuropathy with loss of protective sensation in their feet. Most people with this condition have good blood circulation in their feet.

Your provider may order x-rays or an MRI to look for signs of damage to the bones in your foot and ankle. A bone density scan can measure the strength of your bones, and blood tests can determine if you have an underlying infection.

How Is It Treated?

Medical treatment is directed at taking weight off the foot (*off-loading*), treating bone disease, and healing the wound. Staying off your foot after an injury is the best way to let the bones heal and prevent serious infection. Elevating your foot can help the swelling go down.

While the injury heals, your provider might place your foot in a cast or a removable cast walker. Casts are removed and replaced every few weeks to examine the skin and to adjust for reduced swelling. After the final cast is removed, your provider might prescribe a special brace or custom shoes to accommodate and protect the foot and ankle while the bones and soft tissues continue to heal.

Surgery is sometimes required to treat severe cases of Charcot joint disease. Your health care provider will discuss the best treatment options for your condition.

- A minor foot injury in people with diabetes who have nerve damage in the feet can trigger a cascade of events leading to fractures and dislocations of the bones and joints of the foot. The foot, ankle, or both can subsequently collapse.
- Walking on a deformed foot causes foot ulcers and infections that can lead to amputation.
- Seeking early medical attention at the first sign of a foot injury is important.
- The key to treatment is the prevention of deformity and ulceration. This is achieved by staying off the affected foot and ankle and avoiding further injury until the bones and soft tissues heal.
- Seeing a foot-care specialist, or podiatrist, is often needed for the management of foot complications and regular preventive foot care.

THE MUSCLE, SKIN, AND BONE
Skin Conditions

As the body's largest organ, the skin protects us from germs and harmful elements in the environment; helps regulate body temperature; and allows the sensations of touch, heat, and cold. In some instances, health care providers can diagnose a new case of diabetes or detect complications of the disease in people who have diabetes just by noticing changes in their skin.

▶ WHAT YOU NEED TO KNOW

Skin problems affect many people with diabetes and usually fall into one of several categories.

Autoimmune Responses

Certain skin problems can result from a case of mistaken identity in which the body's immune system gets confused, mistakes itself for a threat, and mounts a defense. Known as an *autoimmune response*, this occurs more often in people with type 1 than type 2 diabetes. For instance, vitiligo is an autoimmune skin condition in which the skin loses patches of color. It occurs more often in people with type 1 diabetes.

Insulin Injection Site Reactions

People who take insulin shots might notice sunken spots (or *lipoatrophy*) due to a loss of fat under the skin, raised and puffy lumps (or *lipohypertrophy*) due

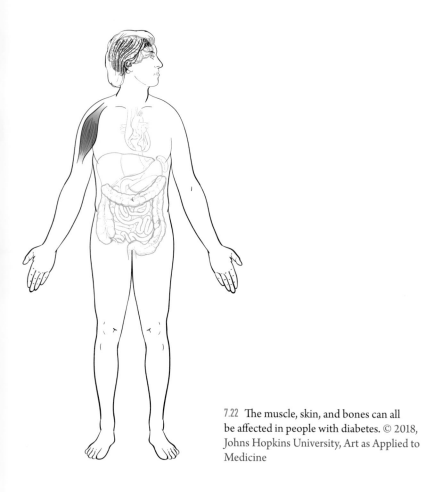

7.22 The muscle, skin, and bones can all be affected in people with diabetes. © 2018, Johns Hopkins University, Art as Applied to Medicine

to the accumulation of fat, and sometimes itchy skin around the injection site. Rotating the site of injection usually helps.

Blisters

People with a long history of diabetes sometimes develop small painless blisters on the hands, feet, or legs (called *diabetic bullae*). These often heal in about a month without requiring treatment.

Digital Sclerosis

Skin that is hard or thickened on the fingers or toes may indicate a condition called *digital sclerosis*. Fingers may become stiff and feel as if there are pebbles in the fingertips. Thickened skin that has the texture of an orange peel can spread to the knees, ankles, and elbows. The legs may become difficult to straighten. People with difficult-to-manage diabetes or complications from diabetes are more likely to develop this skin condition. Physical therapy can help with bending the fingers, toes, or other areas with joints.

Infections

These occur most often in people with poorly controlled blood glucose levels but can affect anyone with diabetes. Two types of infections are the most common: yeast infections and bacterial infections. Areas where the skin rubs together—in the genital and breast areas, for example, or between your toes and around your nails—are prone to yeast infections, which result in itchy, moist skin, and a doughy smell. Any area of the body can develop bacterial infections with red, hot, painful, swollen skin that may develop a white, pus-like discharge. These infections can spread—for example, from a toe to the entire foot—and lead to cellulitis. If treatment is not pursued, these infections can enter the bloodstream and cause a life-threatening condition called *sepsis*. Zygomycete is a rare but life-threatening fungus that can infect the skin of the face and cause fever, blindness, and numbness. This fungus usually targets older people with diabetes.

Chronic Wounds or Ulcers

Open sores or wounds on the foot are called *diabetic foot ulcers* (see "Foot Ulcers" on page 171) and can occur in people with foot deformities, nerve damage, or poor circulation in the feet. These wounds may be associated with an underlying skin infection. Without proper treatment, some chronic wounds or ulcers associated with poor circulation or infections may lead to amputation.

Necrobiosis Lipodica Diabeticorum

This skin condition usually appears on the shins but may also occur on the forearms, hands, and trunk. Usually, there are no symptoms at first except for shiny, red-brown or yellowish skin patches that may gradually become tender and ulcerate. If an injury occurs to the skin in the affected area, it may develop into an ulcer and take a long time to heal. The skin condition occurs more often in women than men and may sometimes be the first presenting symptom of diabetes. However, it does not appear to be related to whether diabetes is well managed or not.

Granuloma Annulare

Pinkish, flesh-colored raised bumps that form ring-shaped patches can appear in people with diabetes. They are more likely than others to develop the rash over large portions of their bodies, including the trunk, arms, and legs. Usually, there are no other symptoms, and the rash disappears after a few months.

Eruptive Xanthomatosis

Small fat-filled blisters can appear on the elbows, buttocks, thighs, or backs of the knees in this condition. When yellowish, scaly patches appear around the eyelids due to high fat levels in the blood, the condition is called *xanthelasma*. These bumps are yellowish in color and are often tender or itchy. When diabetes and cholesterol become better managed, this skin problem usually goes away.

Shin Spots

Brown spots (or lines) on the skin of the knees or lower legs occur in many people with diabetes, more often in men than women, and are called *diabetic dermopathy*.

Velvety Skin

Some people develop dark, velvety patches in folds of skin, usually around the neck, in the armpits, or on the elbows. The condition (*acanthosis nigricans*) itself is harmless, but it is a sign that the body no longer responds well to insulin. This is especially common in people with insulin resistance or type 2 diabetes or women with polycystic ovarian syndrome. Weight loss and dietary changes often help treat this problem.

Skin Tags

People with high insulin levels in the blood (due to insulin resistance) or type 2 diabetes are more likely to develop skin tags, which are growths of skin that hang from a stalk. They occur most commonly on the eyelids, neck, armpits, and groin.

Yellow Nails

Experts still aren't sure why fingernails and toenails turn yellow in some people with diabetes, but this doesn't appear to be a serious problem. The palms of the hands or the soles of the feet sometimes turn yellow too.

Dry Skin

Extremely dry and itchy skin can occur among people with diabetes, particularly if the diabetes is not well managed. If you have autonomic neuropathy or poor blood circulation, you may be more likely to develop dry skin.

Scleredema

Thickening of the skin, called *scleredema*, can occur in patients with diabetes; it is more common in men than women. The skin may feel hard or "woody" in this condition. Typically, the neck and upper back are affected.

- Many people with diabetes have skin problems.
- Your health care provider might refer you to a dermatologist, who can diagnose most problems by taking a close-up look at your skin and prescribe appropriate treatment. In some cases, the dermatologist may remove a small piece of skin, known as a biopsy, and send it off for further testing.
- Infections must be treated quickly to prevent their spread to healthy skin. Your provider might prescribe antibiotics that are taken orally or used in a skin cream. In some cases, hospitalization or surgery might be necessary.
- Check your skin regularly and let your provider know if you notice anything abnormal.

Muscle and Joint Diseases

Aches and pains are common with age, but these issues can signal a serious health problem in people with diabetes. Muscle and joint diseases, also called *musculoskeletal diseases*, affect many people with diabetes.

▶ WHAT YOU NEED TO KNOW

Pain and stiffness in the shoulders, hands, back, hips, knees, and feet are most common, but pain and stiffness can affect any area of the body. If these symptoms persist for longer than a few weeks, your provider might refer you to a specialist, such as a rheumatologist, orthopedic surgeon, or physical therapist.

General Aches and Pains

If multiple joints throughout the body feel painful or stiff, your health care provider might diagnose one of the following conditions:

Osteoarthritis

- This causes joint stiffness and pain, often in the hands, neck, hips, lower back, or knees, and often in people who are overweight.
- Providers usually recommend physical therapy, pain medications (acetaminophen or NSAIDS, such as ibuprofen, if the person does not have kidney disease), topical treatments, injections (steroids or hyaluronic acid), or joint replacement surgery.

Stiff Person Disease

- This causes severe stiffness in the spine, legs, and feet that worsens over time.

- It is a rare neurologic condition and can occur in people with type 1 diabetes.
- Providers usually recommend a regular exercise program combined with medications called *benzodiazepines*.

Diabetic Muscle Infarction

- This is a rare complication of diabetes that destroys muscle tissue because of a lack of blood flow to the area. This usually occurs in the legs and feet. Often only one side of the body is affected.
- Your provider might remove a small section of muscle tissue for further testing before confirming the diagnosis.
- Providers usually treat this condition with rest, pain medications, and drugs that reduce inflammation. Surgery is sometimes considered for severe cases.

Symptoms in the Hands

If pain or stiffness is limited to the hands, one of these conditions could be the reason:

Diabetic Stiff Hand Syndrome

- This condition causes difficulty in the moving joints, particularly the small joints in the hand, making it difficult to flatten the hand.
- Thick, tight, and waxy skin may be present on the back of the hand.
- This condition usually affects older people or those who have had diabetes for many years. Often these people have poor blood glucose management and other health problems related to diabetes, including kidney disease or poor vision.
- Providers usually recommend physical therapy, quitting smoking, and strategies to improve blood glucose management.

Carpal Tunnel Syndrome

- Pain and numbness or tingling in the fingers is sometimes a sign of carpal tunnel syndrome, which occurs due to compression of the median nerve in the wrist. People sometimes notice a weak grip.
- This often occurs after long periods of repetitive movement, such as typing on a keyboard.
- Your provider might rotate or tap on your wrist to see if your pain increases with certain movements. An electrical test of nerve activity in the hand can also confirm the diagnosis.
- Providers usually treat this condition by wrapping the wrist in a splint

when sleeping and usually recommend ibuprofen or other NSAIDS, steroid injections, or surgery.

Dupuytren Contracture

- Many people with diabetes experience stiffness in their hands with no signs of swelling. Some people also see dimples on their palms. These are signs of a condition known as *Dupuytren contracture*.
- Sometimes this condition gets worse with time, but some people find that their symptoms disappear.
- Stretching and massage can help people with mild symptoms. Other people find relief with steroid injections or surgery to release the tense tissue.

Flexor Tenosynovitis

- Some people with diabetes feel stiffness and pain when bending their pointer finger, a condition known as *flexor tenosynovitis*.
- Providers often recommend steroid injections or surgery. Sometimes multiple surgeries are needed to provide relief.

Symptoms in the Shoulders

If pain or stiffness is in the shoulders, one of these conditions could be the reason:

Adhesive Capsulitis

- As many as one-third of people with diabetes lose movement in one shoulder, reporting that the shoulder feels painful and frozen in place. This is known as *adhesive capsulitis* (also commonly called "frozen shoulder"). Though adhesive capsulitis feels like arthritis, the underlying cause is different.
- Older people, those who have had diabetes for many years, and those who have other diabetes-related problems are more likely to develop this condition.
- Providers often recommend physical therapy, steroid injections, and surgical procedures.
- As with many complications, good management of blood glucose can prevent this from occurring.

Calcific Shoulder Periarthritis

- This condition occurs when calcium crystals are deposited in the tissue around the shoulder, causing pain and stiffness in people with diabetes.
- Providers often treat this condition by removing the crystals, injecting steroids, or performing surgery.
- This condition should be distinguished from other more common

medical conditions such as shoulder bursitis (inflammation of the fluid surrounding the joints) and shoulder tendonitis (inflammation of the tendons in the shoulder).

WHAT DOES IT ALL MEAN?

- Diabetes is associated with a number of different muscle and joint problems.
- The hands, neck, shoulders, hips, back, knees, feet, and muscles can all be affected.
- Losing weight, improving blood glucose management, and avoiding cigarettes can help prevent some of these complications; in some cases, medications to reduce inflammation (for example, steroids) are needed.
- Rheumatologists, orthopedic specialists, or physical therapists may help treat some of these conditions.

Osteoporosis

Osteoporosis is a condition in which bones are weaker than normal and easily break. Osteoporosis results from a loss of calcium, minerals, and proteins, which are usually densely packed into healthy bones. This is the most common bone disease and is more common in people with diabetes.

▶ WHAT YOU NEED TO KNOW

Osteoporosis is a silent disease that sometimes goes unnoticed until a fracture occurs. It generally does not cause pain unless it leads to a fracture. Fortunately, you don't need to wait until you break a bone to be diagnosed with bone disease and receive effective treatment.

A dual-energy x-ray absorptiometry (DXA) scan gathers information from x-ray images to measure the density of the calcium and the minerals in your bones. For this reason, the DXA scan is called a *bone mineral density test*.

What Is Osteopenia?

Osteopenia is a state of decreased bone density that is not as severe as osteoporosis but is often a warning sign of impending osteoporosis.

Is Bone Disease Linked to Diabetes?

Yes. People with *type 1 diabetes* are at increased risk of developing osteoporosis. This has special implications for children and teens: eating a healthy diet and controlling blood glucose levels during childhood, when bones are growing the fastest, will help ensure that children with type 1 diabetes reach their expected peak bone density as adults. Unfortunately, about half of all middle-aged people with type 1 diabetes have osteopenia, and a quarter have osteoporosis.

People with type 2 diabetes may have weaker bones but not necessarily osteoporosis. They are actually more likely than others to develop fractures in their bones. This suggests that bone strength is not just related to bone density in people with diabetes but may also depend on the quality and architecture of the bone. Scientists are performing studies to learn more about the link between type 2 diabetes and bone fractures.

How Can I Protect My Bones?

Follow these tips to help your bones stay strong as you age:

- Blood tests can reveal whether your vitamin D levels are healthy. If not, your health care provider might recommend over-the-counter, or in some cases prescription-strength, vitamin D supplements.
- When done on a regular basis, weight lifting, resistance training, walking, stair climbing, and dancing can help strengthen your bones as you age.
- Nothing is more important than treating your diabetes. However, too-low blood glucose levels (hypoglycemia) could cause you to fall and injure yourself. Self-monitor your blood glucose levels as recommended by your health care provider.
- Every day, include 1000 to 1200 mg of calcium in your diet, according to the recommended daily allowances for your age, by eating dairy foods, such as milk, yogurt, or cheese. If needed, calcium supplements (sometimes in combination with vitamin D) may be recommended.
- Seeing clearly and feeling the floor beneath your feet are essential to preventing falls, which can lead to fractured bones. Ask your provider for routine checks of your eyes and nerves. If you have diabetic retinopathy with reduced vision or diabetic neuropathy, you may be more likely to fall and sustain a fracture.
- Turn on lights when walking at night and watch for changes in floor levels.
- Other risk factors for osteoporosis include female sex, older age, thinner body type, white or Asian ethnicity, a family history of osteoporosis, poor eating habits, early menopause and postmenopausal status in women, low testosterone levels in men, lack of exercise, smoking, and alcohol use.

How Is Bone Disease Treated?

If regular exercise, avoiding tobacco and alcohol, vitamin D supplements, and a diet rich in calcium aren't enough to keep your bones strong as you age, a variety of medications are available to help.

Bisphosphonates—such as risedronate (brand name Actonel), alendronate (brand name Fosamax), ibandronate (brand name Boniva), zoledronic acid (brand name Reclast), and similar drugs—are the most commonly used class of medications to treat osteoporosis, though many other options exist. Some of these medications are taken by mouth and some are injectable.

If you have osteoporosis, your provider may recommend repeat DXA scans every 1 to 2 years to see if your current treatment is working.

WHAT DOES IT ALL MEAN?

- Fractures are more common in people with diabetes.
- Bone density may or may not be lower than normal on a DXA scan in people with diabetes, even though bones could actually be weaker.
- It is important for people with diabetes to ensure they are obtaining the recommended daily intakes of calcium and vitamin D to keep bones strong and prevent future fractures.
- Detecting this condition early in those at risk is important to avoid fractures.

Testing for Vitamin D Deficiency

A healthy dose of sunlight to your skin can trigger the body to produce vitamin D, a nutrient that helps build healthy bones. However, many people cannot make enough on their own, and supplementation may be needed. People with diabetes not uncommonly have low vitamin D levels, which render them more vulnerable to osteoporosis (see "Osteoporosis" on page 183) and fractures.

▶ WHAT YOU NEED TO KNOW

Most people produce vitamin D when their skin is exposed to the sun. People who live in northern climates, use sunscreen, or don't go outdoors much may not receive enough sun exposure to produce adequate vitamin D. Others consume the vitamin in foods such as fatty fish and fortified milk. The vitamin is also available in dietary supplements. Ideally, the recommended daily intake of vitamin D is between 600 to 800 IU (international units) of vitamin D each day, with older people aiming for the higher end of this range. Some people might require even higher doses if their vitamin D levels are low. Vitamin D helps the body use calcium from the diet.

Table 7.3. Low levels of vitamin D

<table>
<tr><td colspan="2" align="center">YOU MIGHT HAVE LOW LEVELS OF VITAMIN D
IF YOUR BODY HAS DIFFICULTY . . .</td></tr>
<tr><td>. . . making vitamin D from sunlight</td><td>Affects people with dark skin, the elderly, those with liver disease
Common in winter (staying indoors), summer (heavy use of sunscreen)</td></tr>
<tr><td>. . . absorbing nutrients from food</td><td>Affects people who are obese, people who struggle to eat a balanced diet, and those with gastric bypass weight-loss surgery or other gastrointestinal conditions (such as pancreatitis and celiac disease)</td></tr>
<tr><td>. . . using vitamin D efficiently</td><td>People who take steroids, antiseizure drugs, or HIV drugs may deplete body stores of vitamin D very quickly and have low levels in reserve</td></tr>
<tr><td>. . . with other medical conditions</td><td>Women who are pregnant or breastfeeding; people with osteoporosis (weak bones) and those with certain hormonal conditions, such as hyperparathyroidism, also commonly have vitamin D levels checked</td></tr>
</table>

Unfortunately, many people with diabetes have low levels of vitamin D. People with diabetes and vitamin D deficiencies have a higher risk for broken bones, so it's important to know if you are lacking this important vitamin (table 7.3).

Understanding Your Test Results

Your provider may request a blood test to measure your vitamin D levels. Symptoms of vitamin deficiency, such as bone pain, muscle weakness, or generalized fatigue, may not always be present. Your provider may also order vitamin D levels tested if you have other medical conditions that put you at higher risk of vitamin D deficiency. Depending on the cutoff used, vitamin D sufficiency may be defined as a level greater than 20 or 30 nanograms per milliliter (ng/ml).

How Is Vitamin D Deficiency Treated?

If you have low levels of vitamin D, your provider may recommend a daily multivitamin that contains vitamin D, an oral supplement of vitamin D (such as cholecalciferol), or a prescription form of vitamin D known as ergocalciferol (taken weekly). You may also be prescribed a calcium supplement or referred to a dietitian to discuss your calcium intake.

Your blood test might be repeated after taking vitamin D supplementation for 8 weeks. In most cases, people will see a marked improvement in their vitamin D levels.

WHAT DOES IT ALL MEAN?

- Vitamin D deficiency is common in people with diabetes.
- People with diabetes are at even higher risk of osteoporosis (weak bones) if they have vitamin D deficiency, as well.
- Vitamin D deficiency can usually be corrected with over-the-counter supplements or, if needed, a short course of prescription-strength vitamin D supplements followed by over-the-counter vitamin D supplements to maintain healthy blood levels.

CANCER AND DIABETES
Common Cancers

Uncontrolled cell growth that invades healthy tissue or spreads to other areas of the body is known as *cancer*. Not all tumors are cancerous; tumors that are benign do not spread to other parts of the body. Diabetes is associated with a higher risk of certain types of cancer.

▶ WHAT YOU NEED TO KNOW

Obesity, an unhealthy diet, and a lack of exercise can predispose a person to diabetes and lead to worsening blood glucose levels. Unfortunately, these factors can also increase the risk of certain types of cancer in people with diabetes.

Why Does Diabetes Increase the Risk of Cancer?

The exact reasons for the link between cancer and diabetes remain unclear. However, scientists suspect that elevated levels of insulin (because of insulin resistance, which occurs in types 2 diabetes), which is a hormone that promotes the growth of many tissues, might be related to uncontrollable cell growth in

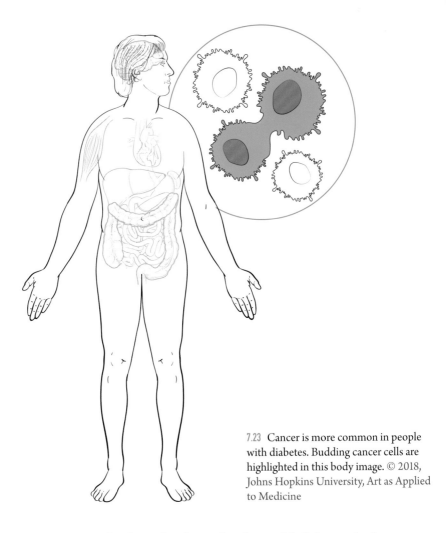

7.23 Cancer is more common in people with diabetes. Budding cancer cells are highlighted in this body image. © 2018, Johns Hopkins University, Art as Applied to Medicine

some cases. Studies have also shown that those with diabetes who have cancer tend to do worse after surgeries and may be more likely to relapse.

Which Cancers Are Linked to Diabetes?

People with diabetes are more likely than others to develop—and die from—non-Hodgkin lymphoma and breast, liver, pancreas, colorectal, and endometrial cancers. The one exception is prostate cancer, which is actually *less* likely to occur in men with diabetes.

Obesity alone has also been linked with higher rates of different types of cancer, too. Interestingly, obese people who undergo bariatric surgery have a reduced risk for these types of cancer.

How Can I Prevent Cancer?

Recent studies suggest that the diabetes medication metformin may lower the risk of some cancers, though scientists are still trying to determine why this is the case.

For now, early detection remains the best way to improve cancer outcomes. People with diabetes should follow the recommended schedule for routine cancer-screening tests, similar to people without diabetes.

WHAT DOES IT ALL MEAN?

- Diabetes and obesity are both linked to an increased risk of many types of cancer.
- Metformin may lower the risk of certain cancers in some studies, but early detection (through appropriate screening) is the best way to improve cancer outcomes.
- Early detection of cancer by following routine preventive screening tests (such as mammogram and colonoscopy) is imperative in people with diabetes.

Pancreatic Cancer

Pancreatic cancer occurs when cells in the pancreas, an organ that sits behind the stomach, begin to multiply rapidly and form a solid mass. Pancreatic cancer is a rare cancer among the general population. People with diabetes are more likely to develop pancreatic cancer, but the overall risk is still very low. Pancreatic adenocarcinoma, the most common type, develops in the parts of the pancreas that do not produce hormones (the exocrine pancreas). Pancreatic neuroendocrine tumors can also sometimes occur in the parts of the pancreas that produce hormones (the endocrine pancreas), but these are extremely rare.

▶ WHAT YOU NEED TO KNOW

Key Facts about Pancreatic Cancer

1 Pancreatic cancer is relatively uncommon, particularly in people younger than 45 years. But as one of the leading causes of cancer-related deaths in the United States, pancreatic cancer can be devastating when it occurs.

2 Many people with diabetes fear they will develop pancreatic cancer, but the risk is relatively low. Though pancreatic cancer is twice as common in people with diabetes, the disease is still relatively rare.

3 Men are more likely than women to develop pancreatic cancer. Smoking,

obesity, a lack of physical activity, an unhealthy diet, and alcohol consumption also increase the risk of developing this disease.

4 Symptoms of pancreatic cancer include abdominal pain, loss of appetite, a yellowish tint to the skin or to the whites of the eyes, unintentional weight loss, bloating, increased belching, an unusual lump in the abdominal area, or sudden difficulties in managing blood glucose.

5 If your health care provider suspects pancreatic cancer, you will likely undergo a CT scan, an MRI scan, or an ultrasound of your pancreas. Your provider may also order blood tests.

6 Because so few people with diabetes develop pancreatic cancer, most providers don't routinely screen for this disease. Your provider might recommend tests for pancreatic cancer if you have any of the symptoms described above.

7 Pancreatic cancer is often diagnosed too late for surgery to help. Pancreatic cancer has typically already spread to nearby organs by the time it is diagnosed. Surgical removal of all or part of the pancreas is often recommended, but not everyone has the disease detected early enough to benefit from surgery. After surgery—or in lieu of surgery—people often undergo radiation therapy, chemotherapy, or a combination of the two. They may also choose not to receive any therapy.

8 Without surgery, people with pancreatic cancer survive an average of 6 to 12 months after diagnosis. Unfortunately, only one-quarter of people survive more than 1 year after diagnosis, and most die within 5 years after diagnosis. Scientists are working very hard to improve the early detection of pancreatic cancer so that in the future, people can be diagnosed earlier and treated more successfully.

WHAT DOES IT ALL MEAN?

- Pancreatic cancer is an uncommon cancer that rarely occurs in younger adults.
- The risk of getting pancreatic cancer is higher among people with diabetes, but overall this risk remains very low.
- Symptoms include abdominal pain, unintentional weight loss, and possibly difficult-to-manage blood glucose levels.
- In very rare cases, diabetes diagnosed later in life (such as over the age of 65) without any other traditional risk factors for diabetes may be an early sign of pancreatic cancer.

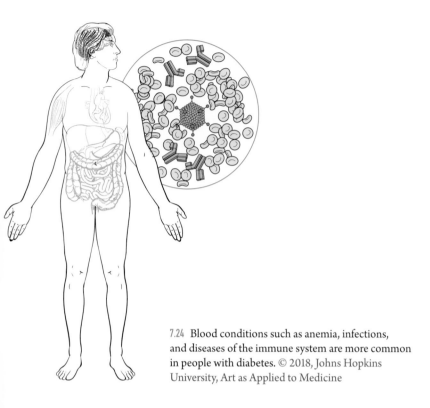

7.24 Blood conditions such as anemia, infections, and diseases of the immune system are more common in people with diabetes. © 2018, Johns Hopkins University, Art as Applied to Medicine

ANEMIA, INFECTIONS, AND THE IMMUNE SYSTEM
Anemia

Anemia is a medical condition marked by having a low red blood count. This condition has many causes and may not lead to any symptoms if mild. However, anemia can result in a number of common symptoms if more severe.

▶ WHAT YOU NEED TO KNOW

Your health depends on red blood cells to carry oxygen from your lungs to the rest of your body. Anemia, a condition in which there are too few red blood cells, can leave you feeling tired and weak.

Anemia can affect anyone. But if you have diabetes, anemia can sometimes hint at problems with your kidneys. A major reason for anemia among people with diabetes is chronic kidney disease. Healthy kidneys produce a hormone called *erythropoietin* (EPO) that stimulates red blood cell production from the bone marrow. EPO may not be produced in sufficient amounts when the kidneys are damaged.

Certain other health issues, mild or severe, can cause anemia. In general, if you have anemia, your body either is not making enough red blood cells (either from nutritional deficiencies or other problems) or is destroying or losing red blood cells at an increased rate. Bleeding may be occurring internally in the stomach or intestines, which can be very slow and not readily detectable. Your provider can gather clues about these underlying causes by having your red blood cells examined under a microscope and sending tests to see whether nutritional deficiencies of iron, vitamin B12 levels, or folate exist. There may also be genetic causes (for example, sickle cell trait or disease). The severity of anemia is determined by performing a complete blood cell test to measure the levels of the iron-rich protein called *hemoglobin*, an oxygen-carrying molecule found in red blood cells.

If these tests show hemoglobin levels lower than 13 (grams per deciliter) g/dL if you are a man or 12 g/dL if you are a nonpregnant woman, you may be diagnosed with anemia. Most cases of anemia are mild or moderate, but hemoglobin levels less than 8 g/dL can be life-threatening and may require more urgent medical treatment, such as a blood transfusion. An alternative measure is hematocrit, which reflects the percentage of blood that contains red blood cells. For adult men, a hematocrit level below 39% is considered anemia. For nonpregnant women, a level below 36% is considered anemia.

Are You at Risk for Anemia?
Your risk of developing anemia is elevated if you:
- are a woman with heavy menstrual bleeding;
- are older in age;
- are a vegetarian or consume a diet low in iron or B vitamins;
- have a gastrointestinal problem, such as a stomach ulcer, other forms of bleeding from the gut, or celiac disease;
- have a weakened immune system due to a short-lived infection or long-term illness, such as an autoimmune disease, a bone marrow disorder, HIV, or cancer; or
- have other health conditions such as sickle cell disease, thyroid disease, or liver disease.

What Are the Symptoms?
It's important to know the possible symptoms of anemia so that you can ask your health care provider for help. Be sure to speak up at your next appointment if you feel very tired, are dizzy, are short of breath, have chronic chest pains, or experience cold hands and feet.

People with mild anemia may not experience any of these signs. But those with severe cases, especially if they are actively bleeding in their guts and are found to have blood in vomit or stool, often have symptoms that require emergency medical treatment.

Your health care provider can order a simple blood test to detect the condition. But be aware that certain factors can interfere with the test results. Dehydration can mask the signs of anemia, so stay hydrated during the hours before your blood draw. Also be sure your diabetes provider knows if you've had a recent blood transfusion because that can alter your results too.

What Is the Treatment?

Iron supplementation is the most common treatment for iron-deficiency anemia. Increasing the dietary intake or taking supplements of folic acid and vitamin B12 may be helpful to keep levels normal. When kidney disease is involved, genetically engineered forms of EPO can be injected to treat anemia. Red blood cell transfusions are sometimes needed in severe cases.

WHAT DOES IT ALL MEAN?

A low level of hemoglobin or hematocrit may indicate that you have anemia. In some cases if you have anemia, your home blood glucose test meter results may not be accurate. A1C results may also be affected by anemia, especially when caused by genetic conditions such as sickle cell disease. Check with your health care provider to find out if abnormal glucose or A1C readings may be related to anemia. Glucose meters are available that provide accurate glucose readings in persons with anemia.

Testing for Autoantibodies

Autoantibody testing refers to laboratory testing to assess the presence of an immune-mediated destruction of the insulin-producing cells of the pancreas. These autoantibodies can cause type 1 diabetes.

▶ WHAT YOU NEED TO KNOW

To understand the concept of an autoantibody, it is important to understand what an antibody is and how it works.

What Is an Antibody?

An antibody is a protein produced by the white blood cells that helps defend the body against potentially harmful foreign substances. You can think of antibodies as soldiers in the body's army, also known as the *immune system*. Antibodies patrol the bloodstream and search for things that don't belong, such as bacteria or viruses. When an antibody encounters a foreign substance, it recruits other members of the army to surround and destroy the "enemy."

What Is an Autoantibody?

An autoantibody is an antibody that gets confused and mistakenly attacks a normal part of the body rather than focusing on foreign substances. In people with type 1 diabetes, autoantibodies attack the cells in the pancreas that produce insulin. The damaged pancreas can no longer produce insulin to lower blood glucose levels, so people with type 1 diabetes must be treated with insulin injections right away.

Are Autoantibodies Produced in Type 2 Diabetes?

People with type 2 diabetes typically do not produce destructive autoantibodies. Instead, the body becomes resistant to the insulin that is produced, and eventually, the pancreas can no longer produce enough insulin to compensate.

How Are Autoantibodies Measured?

Blood tests can detect the following autoantibodies, each of which attacks a different part of the insulin-producing cells in the pancreas:

- Glutamic acid decarboxylase (GAD65)
- Islet antigen-2 autoantibodies (IA-2A)
- Islet cell antibodies (displayed on lab test results as "ICA")
- Insulin autoantibodies (IAA)
- Zinc transporter autoantibodies (ZnT8)

Do Autoantibodies Always Mean That a Person Has Type 1 Diabetes?

Sometimes, people will have autoantibodies in their blood but will not yet have type 1 diabetes. The disease might develop at some point in the future, or the person might never develop the disease. Genetics also appear to play a role, but at this point, it is unclear why some people with autoantibodies develop type 1 diabetes and others do not. Those with more autoantibodies are at increased risk, and everyone with autoantibodies should be followed closely.

Conversely, people who have had type 1 diabetes for many years might gradually have fewer detectable autoantibodies in their bloodstreams. This happens as the pancreas is gradually destroyed.

One or more of these autoantibodies are detected in more than 90% of people with newly diagnosed type 1 diabetes, both adults and children, and can be detected in relatives at risk for developing type 1 diabetes, before clinical onset.

What Can an Autoantibody Blood Test Reveal?

If your health care provider is unsure whether you have type 1 or type 2 diabetes, a blood test can be done to check for autoantibodies. The presence of autoantibodies suggests that a person with elevated blood glucose levels has type 1, rather than type 2, diabetes. This is important to know, as those with type 1 diabetes must always be treated with insulin, whereas those with type 2 diabetes may be managed with oral medications.

Autoantibody testing can be especially useful during pregnancy, as it is sometimes unclear whether a young woman has gestational diabetes (a condition that occurs exclusively during pregnancy) or type 1 diabetes (a long-term condition that does not occur specifically during pregnancy).

If Autoantibodies Are Present, Should Family Members Be Screened?

If a person's blood test shows the presence of autoantibodies in type 1 diabetes, the provider may discuss testing the patient's siblings and children. Often some family members will have autoantibodies but not type 1 diabetes. This indicates that the family members are at a higher risk of developing type 1 diabetes, but they may or may not ever develop the disease.

Useful Facts to Know about Autoantibodies

- More than 70% of people with type 1 diabetes have GAD65 autoantibodies when they are first diagnosed with the disease and before starting insulin therapy.
- The IA-2A test is also very commonly performed.
- The ICA test is the oldest test and is not used as frequently.
- The ZnT8 autoantibody test is the newest and may not be as readily available at all laboratories.
- The IAA autoantibody test looks for antibodies targeting insulin.
- The C-peptide test is commonly performed with autoantibodies. Because levels of this peptide generally match insulin levels in the body, the test can indicate how much insulin your body is producing even if you are being treated with insulin. It is usually low or undetectable in people with type 1 diabetes.

WHAT DOES IT ALL MEAN?

Autoantibodies attack and destroy the body's own insulin-producing cells in the pancreas. People with diabetes and autoantibodies in their blood have type 1 diabetes and will require insulin treatment. Measuring autoantibodies can be a useful tool when the diabetes type is not clear. A negative autoantibody test does not exclude a diagnosis of or future risk for type 1 diabetes.

Infectious Diseases

Infectious diseases are illnesses caused most commonly by viruses, bacteria, and fungi. These occur more often in those with diabetes, particularly those with difficult-to-manage diabetes. Untreated infections in people with diabetes can sometimes lead to severe illness or even death.

▶ WHAT YOU NEED TO KNOW

Does it sometimes seem like you catch every infection that occurs in your school or office? If so, you're not alone. Diabetes increases the chance of having a contagious illness. The most common culprits are the bacteria that cause infections in the legs and feet. People with diabetes are also more likely than others to develop infections after surgery.

Bacteria don't always result in signs or symptoms of infection. For instance, sometimes they are found in the urine without causing noticeable symptoms. But other times, even minor bacterial infections can quickly progress to a serious illness. People with diabetes, for example, are much more likely than other people to die from an infection.

A few infections common in people with diabetes are described below.

Infections of the Genitals and Urinary Tract

People with diabetes are much more likely than others to accumulate high levels of bacteria in their urine. These bacteria don't always cause painful symptoms or progress to a urinary tract infection, but they put these people at higher risk of eventually developing infections. Your health care provider might not prescribe antibiotics unless you have a fever, pain when urinating, or other symptoms of an infection. When antibiotics are prescribed, people with diabetes may need to take the medications for a longer period of time compared with other people. Women with diabetes, particularly if it is poorly managed, may also be more likely to have vaginal yeast infections caused by fungi called *candida*. Both topical and oral antifungal medications are available for treatment of these infections.

Infections of the Legs and Feet

Leg and foot infections, including those that invade the bone (called *osteomyelitis*), are much more common in people with diabetes. If untreated, they can lead to lower limb amputations much more often than in other people. Often these infections start with foot ulcers (see "Foot Ulcers" on page 177).

Respiratory or Lung Infections

The leading cause of pneumonia, in people with and without diabetes, is a bacterium called *Streptococcus pneumoniae*. A vaccine is available to help prevent this type of pneumonia, and all people with diabetes should receive this vaccine at diagnosis and again at age 65, so be sure to ask your health care provider about it. *Streptococcus pneumoniae* causes more severe illness in people with diabetes than without and, if not treated, can be fatal. Be sure to alert your provider if you develop a cough producing green or yellow sputum, along with fever. It is important to catch pneumonia early to prevent poor outcomes.

Influenza, or "the flu," is also a common infection in those with diabetes and can be life-threatening. People with diabetes are much more likely to be hospitalized because of pneumonia from the flu than those without diabetes. A yearly immunization can often help prevent this and is recommended for anyone with diabetes of any age (see "Recommended Vaccinations for People with Diabetes" on page 48).

People with diabetes are also more likely to contract tuberculosis and may be less likely to respond to antibiotics. Though tuberculosis infection can occur in any part of the world, it tends to be more common in developing countries, where the rates of diabetes are also rising and represent a major public health burden.

Skin Infections

These infections, called *cellulitis*, are more common among people with diabetes. They are usually caused by bacteria such as Streptococcus and Staphylococcus. Symptoms include warm, red, swollen, and painful skin. The redness may slowly or rapidly spread. If this happens, seek medical assistance immediately. Antibiotic treatment should be started as soon as possible to prevent the infection from spreading into the bloodstream.

Infection of the Outer Ear

Though infections of the ear canal occur more commonly in those with diabetes, a particularly worrisome infection is *malignant otitis externa*. This is most commonly caused by a bacterium called *Pseudomonas aeruginosa*. People with this condition have a fever along with severe ear pain that sometimes spreads to the face. Urgent medical care is needed to prevent the infection from spreading, as this illness can lead to severe bone and brain complications.

Sinus Infections

Just as in people without diabetes, sinus infections are most often due to bacterial infections in people with diabetes. However, mucormycosis (or zygomycosis) is a rare but potentially severe life-threatening fungal infection that invades blood vessels and can occur more frequently in people with diabetes. In people with very poorly controlled blood glucose levels, if sinusitis does not respond to short-term antibacterial therapy, health care providers may test for zygomycosis.

Taking Antibiotics

If your health care provider prescribes antibiotics for your infection, it is important to use the entire prescription, as directed. Often you will feel better after several days. However, if you stop the antibiotics earlier than prescribed, the infection can come back even stronger. In some instances, infections and sometimes antibiotics may affect blood glucose levels. Be sure to let your health care provider know if your blood glucose levels are too high (or low) when you have an infection.

WHAT DOES IT ALL MEAN?

- People with diabetes are at higher risk for many types of common infections that tend to be more severe and last longer compared to people without diabetes.
- Be sure to notify your health care provider if you develop fever along with any of the symptoms described.
- Antibiotics are sometimes used to treat infections, and it is important to take the entire course of antibiotics prescribed.
- People with diabetes who have poorly controlled blood glucose levels are much more likely to develop infections. Good self-management of blood glucose levels can help prevent future infections from developing.

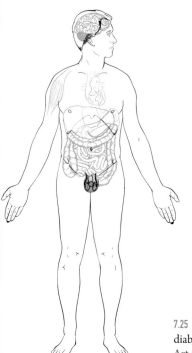

7.25 Men's sexual organs can be affected by diabetes. © 2018, Johns Hopkins University, Art as Applied to Medicine

MEN'S HEALTH
Male Sexual Difficulties

Male sexual dysfunction includes difficulties with sexual interest, erections, ejaculation, and fertility. Such problems are more common in men with diabetes due to the short- and long-term effects of high blood glucose levels.

▶ WHAT YOU NEED TO KNOW

10 Things Men Should Know about Sex and Diabetes

1 Sexual problems affect more than one-third of all men.
2 Men with diabetes are *less* likely than other men to experience satisfying sex lives.
3 Common problems include low sex drive, difficulty reaching orgasm, and early or delayed ejaculation.
4 In addition, some men with diabetes experience erectile dysfunction— trouble getting or keeping a firm erection. This is most common in men with a long history of poorly managed blood glucose levels.

5 Fortunately, many sexual problems have treatments available. These treatments are most successful in men with well-managed blood glucose levels.

6 Erectile dysfunction is not just a sexual problem. It can signal a serious underlying condition, such as nerve damage, low testosterone levels, peripheral and coronary artery disease, or other heart problems.

7 The path to treatment begins in the health care provider's office. Your provider may take your medical history, ask you about your relationship and sexual history, and perform a full physical exam. Some men are referred to a urologist for further treatment.

8 Drugs called *PDE5 inhibitors* (such as sildenafil, vardenafil, tadalafil, and avanafil) are commonly used to treat erectile dysfunction. These drugs cannot be used in men with underlying heart conditions or men taking certain heart drugs (nitrates), some HIV medications (CYP3A4 inhibitors), or specific blood pressure medicines (alpha-adrenergic antagonists). Be sure to ask your provider if you are taking these medications.

9 If PDE5 inhibitors aren't effective, a number of other treatments exist. Some include drugs injected directly into the penis, vacuum suction devices, or prosthetic devices surgically implanted into the penis to help achieve an erection.

10 Psychological counseling can go a long way toward a satisfying sex life. Men can learn self-control techniques to delay ejaculation, recover self-confidence, shed performance anxiety, mend relationship problems, and communicate better with sexual partners. Therapy can also help men address the depression and other mental health issues that often contribute to sexual problems.

WHAT DOES IT ALL MEAN?

Sexual problems occur more commonly in men with diabetes. They may be a sign of poorly controlled diabetes, nerve or blood flow problems, low testosterone, psychological conditions, or heart disease. A careful physical examination and blood work can help identify the cause. Effective treatments are available that can lead to a more enjoyable sex life for men with diabetes who have sexual dysfunction.

Erectile Dysfunction

Erectile dysfunction (impotence) is the inability to get or keep an erection suitable for sexual intercourse and is common in men with diabetes.

MYTH: Men with erectile dysfunction have lost interest in sex.

FACT: Men with erectile dysfunction can have a healthy sex drive but find it difficult to get and keep an erection. Sometimes, however, reduced sexual desire or libido can also occur.

MYTH: Erectile dysfunction only affects a few men with diabetes.

FACT: The majority of older men who have had diabetes for a long time find it difficult to achieve and maintain an erection.

MYTH: Diabetes and erectile dysfunction are completely unrelated.

FACT: Men with diabetes face complications that increase their risk of erectile dysfunction. These include depression, loss of sensation in the penis due to nerve damage, damage to the blood vessels leading to the penis, and reduced levels of a male hormone called *testosterone*. Beta-blockers and other medications for hypertension can also worsen symptoms of erectile dysfunction.

MYTH: Erectile dysfunction is a private matter that doesn't need to be discussed with the health care provider unless the man wants to ask for medication.

FACT: The truth is that men with erectile dysfunction are much more likely to have heart disease. These men are also at risk for complications such as eye damage and nerve damage. Men who have had diabetes for several years—especially those with poorly managed blood glucose levels—face the greatest risk of additional health problems. To effectively monitor for these complications, men should let their health care provider know if they have erectile dysfunction.

MYTH: The only solution to erectile dysfunction is medication.

FACT: Men with diabetes who keep their blood glucose well managed by losing weight, exercising, and eating a healthy diet can sometimes reduce the symptoms of erectile dysfunction. Seeking help for emotional or psychological issues, such as marital problems, depression, and anxiety, can also help with erectile dysfunction symptoms. If lifestyle changes aren't enough, several medications for erectile dysfunction are available, including sildenafil (brand name Viagra), vardenafil (brand name Levitra), tadalafil (brand name Cialis), and avanafil (brand name Stendra). These medications work by boosting blood flow in the penis, making erections easier to get and maintain. Ask your provider which medication would be best for you.

MYTH: Medications for erectile dysfunction always work.

FACT: In some cases, prescription medicines aren't effective. If that happens, the health care provider may refer you to a urologist, a specialist who treats male reproductive conditions. Additional treatments to help a man achieve and maintain an erection include vacuum devices, injectable medications, and surgical implants in the penis.

WHAT DOES IT ALL MEAN?

- Erectile dysfunction is common in men with diabetes and should be discussed with your health care provider.
- Men who take certain medications, including nitrates for heart disease, should not take prescription pills for erectile dysfunction because of potentially dangerous drug interactions. Use with caution when taking alpha-blockers (such as doxazosin) for high blood pressure.
- Consult your health care provider and pharmacist to make sure that pills for erectile dysfunction are safe to take with your other medications.

Low Testosterone (Hypogonadism)

Male hypogonadism is a condition in which the body doesn't produce enough testosterone, the production of sperm is impaired, or both. This can cause many issues in the body, both sexual and nonsexual. Men who have type 2 diabetes, particularly those who are overweight or obese, are more likely to have low testosterone levels. Treatment may be indicated to increase the levels of testosterone in the body.

▶ WHAT YOU NEED TO KNOW

Low testosterone levels may be more common in men who have poorly managed diabetes. Low testosterone levels may also be seen in men who are on chronic opiates or steroids and in those who have other chronic illnesses (for example, kidney or liver failure).

Symptoms

Symptoms of low testosterone may include little or no interest in sex, erectile dysfunction, difficulty concentrating, fatigue, depression, and hot flashes. Men may also experience a decrease in facial or body hair growth, a decrease in muscle size with a gain in fat, and the development of breast tissue. Hypogonadism can cause a low sperm count, leading to difficulties with fertility.

Low testosterone levels may also be associated with a loss of bone mass (see "Osteoporosis" on page 183).

Why Does It Happen?

Male hypogonadism occurs because the testicles do not make enough testosterone. *Primary hypogonadism* refers to a problem in the testicles leading to low testosterone levels. This could occur from a birth defect, a genetic condition, an infection, or exposure to certain cancer treatments, such as chemotherapy and radiation, among other causes.

Secondary hypogonadism refers to a condition in which certain parts of the brain (specifically the pituitary or hypothalamus) do not send enough hormone signals to the testicles to produce adequate testosterone. This can occur because of certain genetic conditions, brain tumors, inflammatory diseases, HIV or AIDS, medications (including but not limited to opiates), aging, illness, or surgery. Secondary hypogonadism is also more common among men with type 2 diabetes or obesity.

Diagnosis

If you have symptoms or signs of hypogonadism, your health care provider may perform a blood test to check your total and free testosterone levels. The best time to check is early, around 8:00 a.m. to 10:00 a.m., since levels fluctuate during the day. If you have a low testosterone level on laboratory tests, it is important to repeat testosterone tests. You need to have at least two low morning testosterone levels before the diagnosis of hypogonadism can be made. After hypogonadism is diagnosed, your provider may order additional blood work (hormonal and nonhormonal) and a semen analysis to help determine the cause of low testosterone. In some situations, a brain MRI may be necessary as well.

Treatment

After you have been diagnosed with hypogonadism, your health care provider may recommend testosterone replacement. Gels or patches applied to the skin or injections (long acting or extra-long acting) are the most common methods to replace testosterone. Less commonly, testosterone pellets may be implanted under the skin, tablets may be applied to the gums, or a specific form of gel may be administered via the nostrils. These medications are not recommended for people with known prostate or breast cancer, severe urinary symptoms, elevated red blood cell count (a hematocrit greater than 50%), untreated severe sleep apnea, high prostate-specific antigen (PSA) levels, or uncontrolled heart failure. The possible side effects of testosterone replacement include enlargement of the prostate; an elevated red blood cell count; rarely, blood clots; acne; breast enlargement; aggressive behavior (more common in teenagers than adults); and worsening of untreated sleep apnea. While some studies have suggested an increased risk of heart attack or stroke in those on testosterone replacement, the data are still unclear and inconclusive.

While you are taking testosterone replacement, your health care provider should closely monitor your testosterone levels, red blood cell count, and PSA laboratory tests, in addition to performing a regular prostate exam.

WHAT DOES IT ALL MEAN?

- Male hypogonadism can cause many symptoms, including fatigue, decreased interest in sex, and difficulties with fertility.
- The diagnosis is based on at least two low-serum-total testosterone levels in the early morning and the symptoms and signs of hypogonadism.
- There are various forms of testosterone replacement. Before starting treatment, it is important to make sure that you do not have other medical conditions in which testosterone treatment would be ill advised.
- It is important to have regular follow-ups with your health care provider and routine blood work while on treatment.

WOMEN'S HEALTH

Pregnancy

Diabetes affects the health of the mother and fetus (the technical term for a baby before it's born) in many ways. Women who have poorly controlled diabetes are at higher risk for miscarriage, stillbirth, premature birth, larger than average babies, and birth defects. The baby may have low glucose levels right after birth, breathing problems, or jaundice (yellowish skin).

▶ WHAT YOU NEED TO KNOW

Fortunately, women with diabetes can take several steps to protect their health and that of their baby before and during pregnancy. If you're planning to get pregnant, work with your doctor ahead of time to get your A1C levels as close to goal as possible. Many experts recommend an A1C goal of less than 6.5% (48 mmol/mol) before getting pregnant. Use effective birth control until your A1C is at goal. Review your medications with your health care provider and

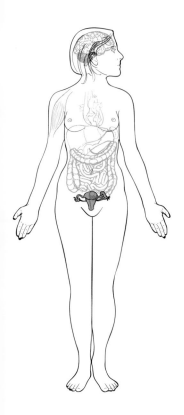

7.26 Women's sexual organs can be affected by diabetes. © 2018, Johns Hopkins University, Art as Applied to Medicine

pharmacist to make sure they will be safe for the baby when you do conceive. Set treatment goals with your provider:

- **For Women with Type 1 Diabetes** Your provider may additionally discuss the use of an insulin pump and continuous glucose monitoring system during pregnancy.
- **For Women with Well-Controlled Type 2 Diabetes or Gestational Diabetes** You may be treated with a low-carbohydrate diet or insulin during pregnancy. Occasionally, oral medications for diabetes may be used. Your health care provider will have you work closely with a dietitian and may refer you to a high-risk obstetrics clinic during pregnancy.
- **For Women with Poorly Managed Type 2 Diabetes** You might require daily insulin injections to control your blood glucose before and during pregnancy.

If you were taking insulin before pregnancy, keep in mind that you may need less insulin early in pregnancy and more insulin than usual later in pregnancy. Immediately after delivery, the insulin requirement decreases dramatically, but your insulin requirements should return to normal within a few days after your baby is born. The abdomen is still a good place for insulin injections during pregnancy. If done correctly, there is no risk to the baby. You may need to check blood glucose levels in the morning upon awakening, before meals, and after meals to get to target.

Remember These Tips

- Blood glucose management is critical before and during pregnancy. Optimal management of your blood glucose levels can dramatically lower the risk of birth defects, premature birth, and stillbirth. Work with your provider to set—and achieve—an A1C goal that's appropriate. Often the A1C goal in pregnancy may be stricter (between 6% to 6.5% or 42 to 48 mmol/mol) than in nonpregnant adults.
- Eye exams may be needed. Get an eye exam before you become pregnant. If you're pregnant, schedule a screening for diabetic eye disease (known as retinopathy), particularly if you haven't had an examination in the past year. Diabetic eye disease may worsen during pregnancy.
- Regular visits during pregnancy are key. Medical tests are performed more often in women with diabetes than in other pregnant women. Your health care provider will monitor your kidney function closely as you and your baby grow, and don't be surprised if you're sent for ultrasounds more often than other pregnant women. Ultrasound images are very helpful in determining when you got pregnant, monitoring the baby's growth, checking for birth defects, and predicting your due date as accurately as possible. Nonstress tests, which monitor whether the baby's heart rate is increasing normally during physical movement, may also be ordered later in pregnancy.

In the Delivery Room

Women who have diabetes will be more carefully monitored during the last few weeks of their pregnancies. When you go into labor, your provider may administer IV insulin to make sure your blood glucose levels are tightly managed during labor and delivery. If ultrasound images suggest your baby is larger than average (over 10 pounds), the provider will likely recommend a cesarean delivery. While a vaginal delivery may be possible, larger babies face a much higher risk of becoming lodged in the birth canal—a life-threatening condition known as *shoulder dystocia*. A scheduled cesarean delivery can avoid this complication and increase the likelihood of a healthy delivery.

WHAT DOES IT ALL MEAN?

If you have diabetes before pregnancy or develop gestational diabetes, tight management of your diabetes is imperative. Keeping glucose levels at goal during pregnancy is critical to protecting the health of both mother and fetus. Preconception counseling, particularly in adolescents with diabetes, can help reduce the risk of complications that may occur with an unplanned pregnancy.

Gestational Diabetes

Gestational diabetes is a type of diabetes that appears specifically for the first time during pregnancy, usually after the 24th week. Though the condition usually resolves after the baby is born, women who develop gestational diabetes face an increased risk of developing the disease again during future pregnancies—and as many as 50% of these women will eventually develop type 2 diabetes in the decade after they give birth.

▶ WHAT YOU NEED TO KNOW

Every year, approximately 1 in 10 expectant mothers develop gestational diabetes. During late pregnancy all women develop some degree of insulin resistance whereby more insulin in the body is required to effectively lower blood glucose levels. However, women who had some insulin resistance before they got pregnant (for example, overweight or obese women) and are unable to produce enough insulin to maintain healthy glucose levels are more likely to develop gestational diabetes later in pregnancy.

Who Is at Risk?

Women are at risk for gestational diabetes if they

- previously had gestational diabetes,
- are overweight or obese,
- have a history of prediabetes (see "Testing for Prediabetes" on page 18),
- have a family history of diabetes in a parent or sibling,
- are older than 25 years of age, or
- belong to a minority racial or ethnic group (that is, African American, Asian American, Hispanic/Latina, Pacific Islander, or American Indian).

Women with gestational diabetes are more likely to have high blood pressure or preeclampsia (dangerously high blood pressure along with protein in the urine and other problems) during pregnancy and to have a cesarean deliv-

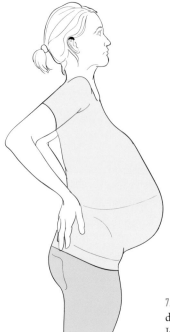

7.27 Women need to be tested for gestational diabetes during the 24th to 28th weeks of pregnancy. © 2018, Johns Hopkins University, Art as Applied to Medicine

ery since the baby may be large (figure 7.27). They are also more likely to be depressed.

How Is It Diagnosed?

Gestational diabetes is most often diagnosed between 24 and 28 weeks of pregnancy. The screening glucose challenge test can be done at any time of the day. Blood glucose is checked 1 hour after drinking a sugary beverage containing 50 grams of glucose. If abnormal, an oral glucose tolerance test must be performed. Alternatively, health care providers may skip the challenge test and order an oral glucose tolerance test from the beginning. For this test women need to be fasting (no food or drink except water for at least 8 hours beforehand), and blood glucose is checked 1, 2, and sometimes 3 hours after drinking a sugary beverage (which contains 75 or 100 grams of glucose). Women at high risk for gestational diabetes may be tested even earlier, at their first prenatal appointment.

How Is Gestational Diabetes Treated?

Keeping blood glucose levels as close to normal as possible without having low blood glucose levels is the goal. Lifestyle changes include the following:

- Undertaking a healthy eating plan and monitoring carbohydrates under the guidance of a dietitian.
- Beginning a daily exercise routine as recommended by the health care provider that is safe during pregnancy.
- If diet and exercise aren't enough, the provider will prescribe insulin injections. Occasionally, oral medications may be used instead.

What to Expect after Delivery

Gestational diabetes typically resolves after the baby is born. Women need to be reevaluated for diabetes at 6 to 12 weeks after delivery. Once blood glucose levels return to normal, women need to be screened for diabetes at least every 3 years because of the increased lifetime risk of developing type 2 diabetes.

WHAT DOES IT ALL MEAN?

Women with gestational diabetes are at an increased risk of developing the condition during future pregnancies and of developing type 2 diabetes during their lifetime. If you have a history of gestational diabetes, ensure that you continue to have regular blood glucose tests after pregnancy. Lifestyle changes, including weight loss, can help reduce the risk of developing type 2 diabetes in the future among women with a history of gestational diabetes.

Female Sexual Difficulties

Female sexual dysfunction may include difficulties with sexual interest, arousal, orgasms, or fertility. Such problems are more common in women with diabetes and may be related to unmanaged diabetes or its complications.

▶ WHAT YOU NEED TO KNOW

10 Things Women Should Know about Sex and Diabetes

1 Sexual problems are twice as likely in women with diabetes than other women.
2 Some women feel low sexual desire, while others have trouble with arousal or orgasm. Pain during intercourse is also more common.
3 These problems happen more often in women with diabetes who have depression or other psychosocial issues.
4 It still isn't clear what causes these problems. Some scientists think hormonal changes might be the reason. Others wonder if weak blood flow to the clitoris might interfere with arousal and lubrication.

There's also evidence that diabetic nerve damage may weaken muscles in the pelvis and vagina and prevent sexual stimulation signals from reaching the brain.

5　While lowering blood glucose levels has many benefits, it remains unclear if this can help prevent female sexual dysfunction. However, too-high or too-low glucose levels at the time of desired sexual activity may interfere with sexual arousal and pleasure and are another reason to strive for good diabetes management.

6　A routine physical exam—including a pelvic exam (performed by a gynecologist), depression screening, and blood tests for hormonal deficiencies or anemia—can help detect underlying health problems. Follow-up care from an endocrinologist can help treat hormonal problems. Women with depression may benefit from counseling.

7　Many women have benefited from lifestyle changes such as exercise and dietary alterations.

8　Estrogen supplements, including low doses applied inside the vagina, may relieve dryness and alleviate pain during intercourse. The oral drug ospemifene (brand name Osphena) has similar benefits to alleviate pain during intercourse by making vaginal tissue thicker and less fragile in postmenopausal women.

9　Diabetes is associated with lower rates of fertility. There are a number of reasons, including weight (for both under- and overweight women), diabetic complications, polycystic ovarian syndrome, and autoimmune destruction of the ovaries (more likely in people with type 1 diabetes). Irregular periods (*oligomenorrhea*) and premature menopause may also contribute to infertility in women with diabetes. However, many women with diabetes are able to conceive successfully, particularly if their diabetes is well controlled and a healthy body weight is maintained.

10　Women who have trouble reaching orgasm have benefited from cognitive behavioral therapy, anxiety-reducing techniques, and education programs designed to teach women how to achieve orgasm.

WHAT DOES IT ALL MEAN?

- Female sexual dysfunction is common in women with diabetes.
- Multiple treatments, including behavior therapy and medications, are available to treat female sexual dysfunction.

Menopausal Effects

Menopause is the phase of life when women stop producing eggs (*ovum*) in their ovaries and cease having menstrual periods. This transition is accompanied by multiple changes in hormones (particularly estrogen), which may affect glucose management in women with diabetes.

▶ WHAT YOU NEED TO KNOW

When a woman's menstrual periods occur less often and have eventually stopped for at least 12 months in a row, she has entered a phase of life known as menopause.

When Does It Happen?

Most women in the United States enter menopause around age 50 years, but women with type 1 diabetes are much more likely to have early menopause (and, because they also have delayed menses, an overall decreased reproductive period of life). Women with type 2 diabetes who are overweight or obese may have later menopause compared to women who are of normal weight or underweight. A woman who has her ovaries surgically removed enters menopause immediately after the procedure. This is called *surgical menopause*.

What Changes Occur?

In the months before menopause, when menstrual periods occur irregularly and further apart, women with diabetes can experience mood swings and may have greater difficulty managing their blood glucose levels due to hormonal changes. Hot flashes and vaginal dryness are also common during this transition. Women with diabetes tend to have worse hot flashes, vaginal dryness, and other symptoms of menopause compared with women who do not have diabetes. Sleeping difficulties due to night sweats may also occur.

These hormonal changes also can cause body fat accumulation around the waistline, resistance to insulin, and increases in bad cholesterol along with decreases in good cholesterol. Regardless of whether a woman has diabetes, menopause increases her risk of heart disease. Diabetes further increases this risk, emphasizing the need for heart disease prevention.

Osteoporosis, a condition resulting in weakening of the bones, occurs much more commonly after menopause. This condition raises the chance of having a fracture. Older women with diabetes are much more likely to have osteoporosis and fracture their hips compared with women who do not have diabetes.

Treatment

Women who experience severe hot flashes or vaginal dryness are sometimes given drugs containing the hormone estrogen, the main female sex hormone, which the body stops producing after menopause. This treatment, known as *hormone replacement therapy*, can paradoxically increase the risk of heart attack and stroke in women if taken for a long period of time and at high doses. However, if the symptoms of menopause are severe, a woman and her provider might discuss the benefits of short-term estrogen therapy with or without other hormone replacement.

Severe symptoms of menopause can sometimes be controlled with prescription medications that do not involve hormones, such as SSRIs (medications typically used for depression), gabapentin, or clonidine. Other options include vaginal moisturizers and other topical lubricants to help relieve vaginal dryness.

To reduce the risk of osteoporosis after menopause, ask your health care provider about routine bone density screening and recommendations for exercise and your daily intake of vitamin D and calcium.

WHAT DOES IT ALL MEAN?

- Menopause leads to changes in hormones and excess body fat that may affect blood glucose levels.
- Treatments exist to lessen the severity of symptoms from menopause.
- Talk to your provider about ways to reduce the risk of heart disease and osteoporosis after menopause.

Menstrual Cycle Effects

Women with diabetes may notice that their blood glucose level changes just before their menstrual cycle starts. Conversely, high blood glucose levels can lead to irregular periods (menses). Anticipating these potential changes can lead to better glycemic management and more predictable menses.

▶ WHAT YOU NEED TO KNOW

A normal menstrual cycle lasts, on average, 28 days from the beginning of one period to the beginning of the next—but nearly a quarter of all women with diabetes will have abnormally short or long cycles or go several months without having a period.

Irregular menstrual cycles have different forms:

- If your period lasts excessively long (over 7 days) with heavy bleeding, your provider might say that you have *menorrhagia*.
- If your cycle is longer than 35 days (that is, you have menstrual periods every 35 days or more), you might be told that you have *oligomenorrhea*.
- When a woman who has always had a regular cycle goes for more than 6 months without having a period, this is known as *secondary amenorrhea*.

Menstrual irregularities can occur regardless of the type of diabetes you have. Teenagers with type 1 diabetes may get their periods later than other girls their age. Later in life, women with poorly controlled type 1 diabetes tend to reach menopause at an earlier age than other women. Abnormal cycles occur most often in women who have high blood glucose levels. Women with type 2 diabetes may find that their periods are shorter and farther apart, compared with a normal 28-day cycle.

Irregular menstrual cycles can cause anxiety in women who are trying to avoid pregnancy and make it more difficult for women to conceive. If you have irregular cycles, work with your provider to set a reasonable goal for blood glucose levels. Even if improving your A1C level does not return your menstrual cycles to normal, it will certainly be favorable to your baby's health if you conceive. If you're trying to avoid pregnancy, ask your doctor whether birth control pills can help you achieve predictable 28-day cycles.

If you take insulin, you might find you need to adjust your dose during the days leading up to your menstrual period. Blood glucose levels are sometimes higher than normal around ovulation—in fact, some women can predict the day they ovulate by the rise in blood glucose. When you test your blood glucose at home, try to notice the patterns that occur every month so that you can talk to your provider about adjusting your insulin accordingly. In contrast, some women experience lower blood glucose levels during their periods. For women who manage diabetes using an insulin pump, consider setting temporary basal rates to help maintain better blood sugar control during this time.

WHAT DOES IT ALL MEAN?

- Menstrual irregularities are common in women with type 1 or type 2 diabetes.
- Achieving better glucose management may help better regulate menses.
- Women may have higher blood glucose levels just before their menses, and those on insulin therapy may need increased medication doses.

Polycystic Ovarian Syndrome

Women with *polycystic ovarian syndrome* (PCOS) may have higher androgen levels (that is, male hormones such as testosterone) than other women. The cause of PCOS is unknown but may be due to a combination of genetics and other issues (such as body weight or environmental factors). Women with PCOS are more likely to develop prediabetes and type 2 diabetes.

▶ WHAT YOU NEED TO KNOW

PCOS is a common hormonal disorder that affects up to 10% of women.

Symptoms

Women with PCOS may have irregular or absent periods and may have multiple small cysts on their ovaries. As a result, women with PCOS may have a more difficult time becoming pregnant spontaneously. Other symptoms of PCOS may include excess growth of dark or coarse hair on the face, chest, and back (called *hirsutism*); acne; and male-pattern hair loss. Some women may also notice darkening of the skin in areas such as the nape of the neck or underarms.

Other Common Health Conditions in Women with PCOS

Many women with PCOS are overweight or obese. Women with PCOS are at increased risk of health problems such as type 2 diabetes and sleep apnea. Even women of normal weight may have insulin resistance (that is, when the body cannot respond to insulin properly) and are at higher risk of developing prediabetes and diabetes. High blood pressure and high cholesterol may also be present. All these conditions together may increase the risk of cardiovascular disease. Women with PCOS may also be at increased risk of endometrial cancer (cancer of the uterus) due to multiple factors such as obesity, diabetes, or problems with ovulation.

Diagnosis

There is no single test for PCOS, and the diagnosis is usually made on the basis of symptoms; physical examination; blood work; and, if needed, ultrasound of the ovaries. To make the diagnosis, your health care provider can perform a thorough exam to check for excess hair growth and blood tests to check the level of testosterone in your body. Sometimes an ultrasound is used to check for cysts on your ovaries. Your provider will also investigate other possible reasons for an irregular menstrual cycle, ranging from pregnancy to hormonal disorders of the endocrine system.

Treatment

- The first treatment is weight loss in women who are overweight or obese. Weight loss (a goal of about 5% to 7% of body weight) is most commonly achieved through healthy eating and physical activity. Losing weight can improve blood glucose levels, reduce the production of testosterone, restore fertility, and promote regular menstrual periods. If weight loss isn't enough to reverse the symptoms of PCOS or if a woman with PCOS is not overweight, a variety of medications are available. These medications should be taken only in consultation with a health care provider.
- Hormonal contraception (for example, birth control pills, skin patch, or vaginal ring) that contains the hormone estrogen or progesterone can reduce excess facial and body hair growth, improve acne, make periods more regular, and potentially reduce the risk of endometrial cancer.
- Spironolactone (see "Diuretics" on page 276) is a blood pressure medication that also partially blocks the effects of excess male hormones (such as testosterone) and can be used to control abundant hair growth and acne if oral contraceptives are not effective. However, this drug can cause harm to a fetus and thus cannot be used during pregnancy.
- Of note, excess hair growth can also be treated by laser hair removal and electrolysis. Over-the-counter facial hair removal creams and prescription creams such as eflornithine (brand name Vaniqa) may slow hair growth.
- Metformin (see "Metformin" on page 225), a medication commonly used for diabetes, is often prescribed to women with PCOS who typically also have insulin resistance or prediabetes. Metformin may help make menstrual periods more regular but is not as effective in controlling body hair.
- Clomiphene citrate and letrozole (used off-label) are drugs that can help women with PCOS ovulate to become pregnant.

WHAT DOES IT ALL MEAN?

- PCOS is a common hormonal condition in women causing high levels of androgens, irregular menstrual periods, and possibly multiple cysts on the ovaries.
- Women with PCOS can have excess hair growth on the face or body and higher rates of infertility (that is, more difficulty getting pregnant).
- Women with PCOS are also often more likely to have prediabetes or diabetes, obesity, high cholesterol, and a higher risk of cardiovascular disease.
- Weight loss in women who are overweight or obese is an important and effective treatment. Many medications also exist to successfully treat symptoms and help achieve pregnancy.

Chapter 8

AN OVERVIEW OF TREATMENTS FOR TYPE 1 AND TYPE 2 DIABETES

Type 1 Diabetes: Insulin Treatment

In type 1 diabetes, the insulin-producing cells in the pancreas are completely damaged by autoantibodies (proteins inappropriately directed against the body). For that reason, persons with type 1 diabetes do not produce any insulin on their own. Every person with type 1 diabetes depends on daily insulin treatment to survive. Insulin can be injected using a vial and syringe (figure 8.1) or pen (figure 8.2), inhaled, or delivered through an insulin pump.

▶ WHAT YOU NEED TO KNOW

What Types of Insulin Are Available?

Two major types of insulin are used to treat people with type 1 diabetes: a) short- or rapid-acting insulin, and b) intermediate- or long-acting insulin (table 8.1). Inhaled insulin (brand name Afrezza) is also available and is similar in effect to rapid-acting insulins. A complete list of insulins available in the United States is provided in the appendix.

Recommended Treatment Schedule

Many people with type 1 diabetes are treated with *intensive* or *basal-bolus* insulin injection therapy, which requires four to six injections a day (one to two injections of basal insulin and three to four injections of bolus insulin before meals and snacks). This method allows a great deal of flexibility with regard to the types of food you eat, when you eat, and how much you eat. Insulin pumps (see "Using an Insulin Pump to Manage Diabetes" on page 296) are an alterna-

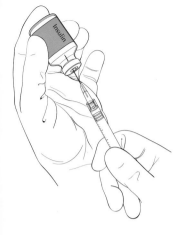

8.1 When using insulin from a vial, a syringe is used to draw up and inject the insulin. © 2018, Johns Hopkins University, Art as Applied to Medicine

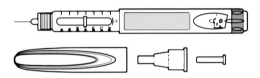

8.2 When using a pen prefilled with insulin, a dose is usually chosen by rotating the dial, and insulin is injected through a needle attached to the pen. © 2018, Johns Hopkins University, Art as Applied to Medicine

tive treatment in which rapid-acting insulin (or sometimes short-acting insulin) is continuously delivered through a catheter under the skin. Inhaled insulin (see "Inhaled Insulin" on page 257) is also an option. Here's how it works:

- The long-acting (basal) insulin is typically taken at bedtime, in the morning, or both.
- Nutritional (bolus) insulin is taken before each meal (and snacks), based on how many carbohydrates are in the food, in addition to correctional (bolus) insulin, which is based on the blood glucose reading before the meal.
- Meeting with a dietitian can help people with type 1 diabetes learn carbohydrate counting, with specific dosing recommendations from the health care provider.
- Self-monitoring of blood glucose is particularly important for persons treated with insulin. Blood glucose can be monitored using a home blood glucose meter, a continuous glucose monitor, or both.

Table 8.1. Types of insulin

TYPE OF INSULIN	EXAMPLES	WHAT THEY DO	WHEN THEY'RE TAKEN
Intermediate- or long-acting (basal) insulin	Glargine (brand names Lantus or Basaglar) or degludec (brand name Tresiba) is usually given once a day Detemir (brand name Levemir) is usually given twice a day in type 1 diabetes and once or twice a day in type 2 diabetes NPH insulin (brand names Humulin N or Novolin N) is usually given twice a day in type 1 diabetes and once or twice a day in type 2 diabetes	Basal insulin keeps blood glucose in a normal range throughout the day, even when the person is not eating	Once or twice a day, depending on which type is prescribed
Short-acting and rapid-acting (bolus) insulin	Short-acting: regular (brand names Novolin R or Humulin R) Rapid-acting: lispro (brand names Humalog or Admelog), aspart (brand names Novolog or Fiasp), glulisine (brand name Apidra)	Nutritional insulin helps the body process carbohydrates from meals Correctional insulin corrects high blood glucose levels before meals	Usually three times a day before meals

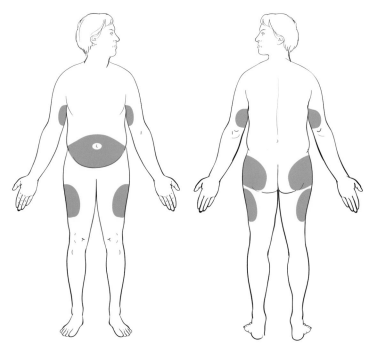

8.3 Common sites for insulin injection include the abdomen, buttocks, upper outer thighs, and upper outer arms. © 2018, Johns Hopkins University, Art as Applied to Medicine

- Common insulin injection sites include the abdomen, buttocks, upper outer thighs, and upper outer arms (figure 8.3). It is important to rotate injection sites to avoid scar tissue forming under the skin, which may affect insulin absorption over time.

WHAT DOES IT ALL MEAN?

People with type 1 diabetes need lifelong insulin therapy that can be delivered through multiple daily injections or an insulin pump. Many different types of insulins are available, with different durations of action. Basal insulins have a long-lasting continuous effect and keep the blood glucose in a healthy range even when the person is not eating. Bolus insulins last for only a few hours and are taken before meals, act quickly, and counteract the glucose spikes that occur with eating. A combination of both basal and bolus insulins is needed to effectively treat type 1 diabetes.

Type 2 Diabetes: Non-insulin Treatment

If you have been diagnosed with type 2 diabetes, chances are your health care provider has recommended weight loss and lifestyle changes, such as a healthy eating plan and regular exercise, to improve your blood glucose control. Your provider will also have likely prescribed metformin when you were diagnosed. When other diabetes medications are needed, providers generally follow a series of steps to choose the best treatment for you.

▶ WHAT YOU NEED TO KNOW

Step 1: Know Your Goals

Your provider can help you set personalized goals. For most nonpregnant adults, the goal A1C level is lower than 7% or 53 millimoles per mole (mmol/mol). Younger adults who have just been diagnosed may have an A1C goal of lower than 6.5% (48 mmol/mol) to reduce their chances of developing long-term complications. Older, frail adults with multiple health problems and physical disabilities might have a goal A1C closer to 8% (64 mmol/mol). As you work toward your goal, be sure to tell your provider if you experience any episodes of high or low blood glucose. A1C goals are individualized and decided between you and your health care provider.

Step 2: Keep Up the Hard Work

Continue to eat a balanced diet and exercise regularly. Healthy lifestyle changes are key in people with type 2 diabetes at all stages and can help medications for diabetes work more effectively or reduce the need for additional medications in the future.

Step 3: Metformin Can Help

The diabetes drug metformin (see "Metformin" on page 225) is often the first medication a health care provider will prescribe for a person with type 2 diabetes. It is one of the oldest drugs for diabetes and is safe, inexpensive, usually well tolerated, and effective—lowering the A1C by up to 1.5% (17 mmol/mol). People with type 2 diabetes typically start on a low dose at the time of diagnosis and work their way up to an appropriate dose that helps lower their blood glucose levels, as long as there are no side effects.

Step 4: When Metformin Isn't Adequate, Other Medications Can Help

People with persistently high blood glucose levels, or those who sometimes cannot tolerate the side effects from metformin, often require a second or third type of medication in addition to or instead of metformin. If you're one of those people, your health care provider will choose among several available medications to find the best treatment based on your medical history. Many classes of oral medications are available, and a complete list is provided in the appendix. Each of these classes of medicines works to lower glucose in a different way. These include

- *sulfonylureas*, such as glyburide (brand name DiaBeta Micronase, Glynase), glipizide (brand name Glucotrol), and glimepiride (brand name Amaryl);
- *meglitinides*, such as nateglinide (brand name Starlix) and repaglinide (brand name Prandin);
- *thiazolidinediones*, such as pioglitazone (brand name Actos) and rosiglitazone (brand name Avandia);
- *alpha-glucosidase inhibitors*, such as acarbose (brand name Precose) and miglitol (brand name Glyset);
- *DPP-4 inhibitors*, such as sitagliptin (brand name Januvia), saxagliptin (brand name Onglyza), linagliptin (brand name Tradjenta), and alogliptin (brand name Nesina); and
- *SGLT2 inhibitors*, such as canagliflozin (brand name Invokana), dapagliflozin (brand name Farxiga), and empaglipflozin (brand name Jardiance);
- additionally, some medications commonly used in other conditions can also treat type 2 diabetes, including bromocriptine (brand name Cycloset) and colesevelam (brand name Welchol).

Non-insulin injectable medications are also available:

- *GLP-1 receptor agonists*, such as exenatide (brand name Byetta or Bydureon), liraglutide (brand name Victoza), dulaglutide (brand name Trulicity), lixisenatide (brand name Adlyxin), and semaglutide (brand name Ozempic)
- *Amylin analogs*, such as pramlintide (brand name Symlin)

Step 5: Insulin Injections Are Always an Option

If you've tried multiple pills or non-insulin injectables without successfully lowering your blood glucose levels to goal, your provider may suggest starting with a single daily injection of insulin in addition to your other medicines and then increasing the frequency of injections as needed.

Persons who take insulin must continue to monitor their blood glucose levels closely to adjust treatment and avoid low blood glucose levels. Oral medications for diabetes may need to be continued, reduced, or stopped completely once insulin is started.

Multiple medications are available to treat type 2 diabetes along with lifestyle changes. The choice of medication depends on many factors, such as its effectiveness in lowering blood glucose levels, its cost, its changes to body weight, its risk for too-low blood glucose levels (hypoglycemia), and its side effects. Metformin is commonly used as the first drug treatment, but multiple medications may be required to treat diabetes over time. In people with a history of cardiovascular disease (such as heart attacks or stroke), specific medications that have additional cardiovascular benefits may be preferred as the next step. When oral medications or non-insulin injections are no longer able to lower blood glucose levels, insulin therapy may be needed. Type 2 diabetes is a progressive disease, and even if you do everything right, you may still need higher doses or more medications over time. Needing to add insulin therapy is not a sign of failure. Talk to your health care provider about the best treatment for your diabetes.

Type 2 Diabetes: Insulin Treatment

The decision to take insulin is never an easy one. For many people it comes after years of having type 2 diabetes and trying multiple weight-loss regimens, diets, and oral medications. For other people the decision to take insulin is made sooner after diagnosis or when blood glucose levels are simply too high to manage with other drugs.

▶ WHAT YOU NEED TO KNOW

The good news is that insulin should always work when given in the correct doses. Daily injections can be very effective at managing blood glucose levels. Anxious about giving injections? Help is available. If your health care provider prescribes insulin, a trained diabetes educator or pharmacist can teach you how to measure out the proper dose and administer your daily injections.

Why Should I Use Insulin?

With type 2 diabetes, over time the pancreas "burns out" and is only able to produce small amounts of insulin—this is the progressive nature of the disease. When this happens, your blood glucose levels will become very difficult to manage without daily injections of insulin. Injectable insulin is similar to that made by the body but can be categorized into two main types: basal insulin and bolus insulin. Basal insulin (long-acting and intermediate-acting insulin) keeps your blood glucose stable all day long, even when not eating. Bolus insulin (rapid-acting and short-acting insulin) helps your body respond to the quick rise in blood glucose after meals.

The insulins used to treat type 2 diabetes are the same as those used for the treatment of type 1 diabetes. However, persons with type 2 diabetes might take insulin therapy anywhere from one to four times a day, depending on their needs, and usually do not need insulin at diagnosis. In contrast, those with type 1 diabetes usually take insulin therapy four times a day and will always require insulin treatment from the time they are diagnosed.

Another key difference is that persons with type 2 diabetes often require much higher doses of insulin than those with type 1 diabetes due to their body's inability to respond to insulin and effectively lower blood glucose (also called *insulin resistance*). As a result, more concentrated insulins may be recommended to reduce the volume of insulin given with each injection for those with type 2 diabetes on high doses. The standard insulin concentration is U-100, which represents 100 units of insulin per milliliter. The concentrated insulins currently available include

- U-200 lispro insulin (brand name Humalog),
- U-500 regular insulin (brand names Novolin R or Humulin R),
- U-300 insulin glargine (brand name Toujeo), and
- U-200 insulin degludec (brand name Tresiba).

In comparison to U-100 insulin, U-200 insulin has 200 units of insulin per milliliter (two times more concentrated), U-300 insulin has 300 units of insulin per milliliter (three times more concentrated), and U-500 insulin has 500 units of insulin per milliliter (five times more concentrated). Dose changes are sometimes needed when switching from the standard U-100 insulin to more concentrated insulins.

Who Needs Insulin?

You might need insulin therapy if

- you have trouble managing your blood glucose with diet and exercise despite multiple oral or non-insulin injectable diabetes medications,
- your A1C level is higher than 10% at diagnosis (86 mmol/mol) or your blood glucose level is higher than 300 milligrams per deciliter (mg/dL) or 16.7 millimoles per liter (mmol/L) at any time of day,
- you have side effects with other diabetes medications and continue to have poorly managed blood glucose, or
- you often experience thirstiness, frequent urination, or other symptoms of high blood glucose despite taking other medications.

WHAT DOES IT ALL MEAN?

- Over time most people with type 2 diabetes will eventually require insulin treatment. Insulin may be needed anywhere from a few years to many decades after being diagnosed with type 2 diabetes. The timing is different for each person.
- Other diabetes medications, such as oral medications or non-insulin injectable medications, are sometimes continued when insulin is started, but the doses may need to be reduced.
- Some people with type 2 diabetes and everyone with type 1 diabetes need to be on insulin treatment right away.

Chapter 9

MEDICATIONS COMMONLY USED TO TREAT DIABETES

PILLS AND NON-INSULIN INJECTABLE MEDICATIONS
Metformin

Metformin belongs to a class of medications called *biguanides* and is commonly recommended as the first medication for people with type 2 diabetes who do not have any contraindications. In addition, it is sometimes used to prevent diabetes in people who are at risk of developing the disease, such as those with prediabetes but is not currently FDA-approved for this condition. Many people find that their A1C levels drop, on average, by 1% to 1.5% or 11 to 17 millimoles per mole (mmol/mol) on this medication alone. It can be taken with other oral diabetes medications, non-insulin injectable medications, and insulin.

▶ WHAT YOU NEED TO KNOW

What Is Metformin?

Metformin is manufactured under several different brand names. These are the most common:

- Metformin hydrochloride (brand name Glucophage, but also a common generic medication)
- Metformin ER (extended release; brand name Glucophage XR, Glumetza, and Fortamet)

What Does It Do?

Metformin primarily reduces the liver's tendency to release stored glucose (glycogen) into the blood when it is not needed (figure 9.1).

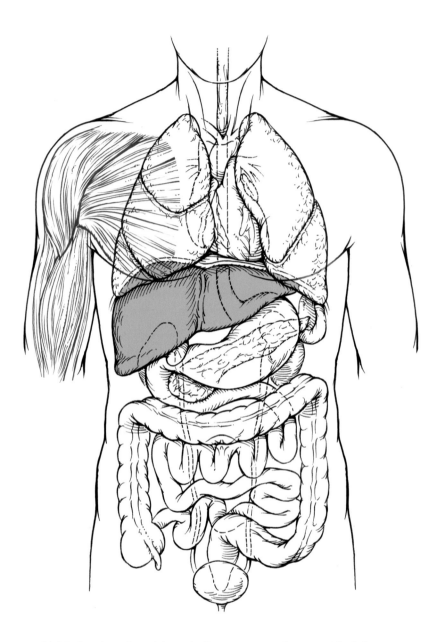

9.1 Metformin works mainly on the liver, an organ in the upper right abdomen, to increase insulin sensitivity. Metformin prevents the liver from breaking down glucose stores (*glycogen*) and releasing glucose into the bloodstream. Metformin may also increase the sensitivity of skeletal muscle to insulin.

How Is It Taken?

Metformin is usually taken with meals either once or twice a day depending on the brand. Available dosages of pills include 500 milligram (mg), 750 mg, 850 mg, and 1000 mg.

The treatment plan will differ for each person, but a common starting regimen is listed below:

- To avoid stomach upset, people usually start with a very low dose (500 mg) taken with dinner.
- After a few weeks or so, the dose may increase to 500 mg with breakfast and 500 mg with dinner.
- A few weeks later, the dose may increase again to 500 mg with breakfast and 1000 mg with dinner.
- If the person has no side effects, the dose may increase to 1000 mg with breakfast and 1000 mg with dinner. This is usually the maximum dose. Sometimes, with the 850 mg pill, the maximum daily dose can go up to 2550 mg daily.
- Several types of combination pills are available that include metformin and other diabetes medications together in one tablet (see the appendix).

Facts about Metformin

1 Metformin is the treatment of choice for type 2 diabetes because it works very well in lowering blood glucose, is safe, is inexpensive, and has been around for decades.
2 People with diabetes may lose a few pounds of weight on metformin.
3 By itself metformin does not usually result in too-low blood glucose levels (hypoglycemia).
4 Common side effects include nausea and diarrhea. However, taking metformin with food, slowly increasing doses, or using extended release preparations can often prevent them.
5 In rare cases, metformin can have a serious side effect called *lactic acidosis*, where the body produces potentially dangerous levels of lactic acid. This condition is rare and occurs more commonly in persons who are older or have severe heart failure, a history of heavy alcohol use, or advanced kidney or liver disease.

Warning!

- People with advanced liver or kidney problems may need to take reduced doses of metformin or discontinue this medication.

- Pregnant women should talk to their providers before taking this medication. In some women metformin may be safe to take during pregnancy.
- People generally should *not* take metformin immediately before—or 48 hours after—receiving intravenous (IV) contrast for a CT scan.
  As a result, metformin is often stopped temporarily when a person is hospitalized.

WHAT DOES IT ALL MEAN?

- Metformin is the most commonly prescribed first medication for newly diagnosed persons with type 2 diabetes who do not have extremely high blood glucose levels. It has a moderate effect on lowering blood glucose levels by decreasing A1C 1% to 1.5% (11 to 17 mmol/mol).
- A liquid solution of metformin (brand name Riomet) is also available for people who have difficulty swallowing pills.
- While usually well tolerated, gastrointestinal side effects, such as diarrhea, can occur.

Alpha-Glucosidase Inhibitors

Alpha-glucosidase inhibitors are recommended for people with type 2 diabetes who have high blood glucose levels despite using other medications for diabetes. These are typically not first-line treatments but may be used as additions in persons with diabetes who are already using other therapies. On average, most people find that their A1C levels drop by approximately 0.5% to 1% (5.5 to 11 mmol/mol) on these medications.

▶ WHAT YOU NEED TO KNOW

What Are Alpha-Glucosidase Inhibitors?
Two alpha-glucosidase inhibitors are available:
- Acarbose (brand name Precose)
- Miglitol (brand name Glyset)

What Do They Do?
These pills work in the gut by slowing the digestion and absorption of sugars from meals. This is accomplished by blocking an enzyme known as *alpha glucosidase*, which normally helps the body break down carbohydrates into simple sugars that can be absorbed through the small intestine (figure 9.2).

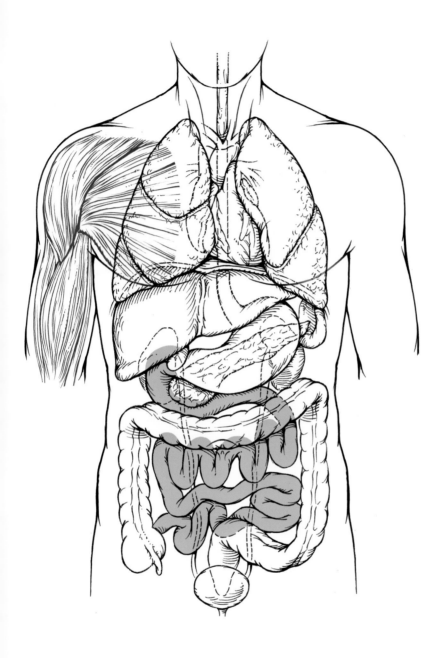

9.2 Alpha-glucosidase inhibitors work in the small intestine, preventing the breakdown and absorption of carbohydrates from ingested food. © 2018, Johns Hopkins University, Art as Applied to Medicine

How Are They Taken?

Acarbose and miglitol are taken at the beginning of meals. The treatment plan will differ for each individual but in general:

- Acarbose or miglitol is taken three times a day; the health care provider may gradually increase each dose from 25 mg to as much as 100 mg three times a day with meals.

Facts about Alpha-Glucosidase Inhibitors

1 People generally don't gain or lose weight on these medications.
2 When taken alone, these medications do not cause low blood glucose.
3 Common gastrointestinal side effects of these drugs include gas, diarrhea, bloating, and abdominal cramps, especially when used with a high-carbohydrate diet.

Warning!

- Pregnant women should talk to their providers before taking this medication.

WHAT DOES IT ALL MEAN?

- Alpha-glucosidase inhibitors are given in pill form.
- Gastrointestinal side effects are common, which may limit their use.
- These medications have a mild effect on lowering blood glucose levels (A1C lowering of about 0.5% to 1% or 5.5 to 11 mmol/mol) and can be used as add-on therapies to other medications for diabetes.

DPP-4 Inhibitors

DPP-4 inhibitors are a class of oral diabetes medicines used to treat people with type 2 diabetes. DPP-4 inhibitors are recommended for people with type 2 diabetes who have high blood glucose levels. On average, most people find that their A1C levels drop by 0.5% to 1% (5.5 to 11 mmol/mol) on these medications.

▶ WHAT YOU NEED TO KNOW

What Are DPP-4 Inhibitors?

These medications are available as oral tablets. Several DPP-4 inhibitors are available commercially. The following provide some examples:

- Sitagliptin (brand name Januvia)

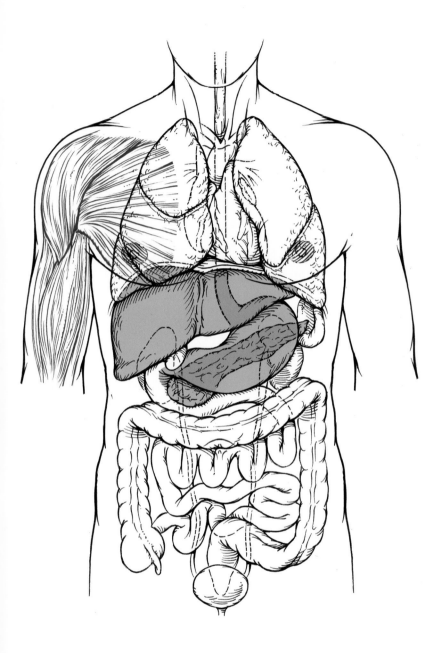

9.3 DPP-4 inhibitors have effects on the liver (preventing glucose release), stomach (slowing food emptying), and pancreas (helping more insulin to be released when food is eaten), which together result in a lowering of blood glucose levels. © 2018, Johns Hopkins University, Art as Applied to Medicine

- Saxagliptin (brand name Onglyza)
- Linagliptin (brand name Tradjenta)
- Alogliptin (brand name Nesina)

Many of the DPP-4 inhibitors are also sold in a pill combined with metformin (see the appendix).

What Do They Do?

These medications prevent the breakdown of a hormone released by the gut, called *GLP-1*, that stimulates the pancreas to release insulin, slows food leaving the stomach, and blocks the breakdown of glycogen from the liver (figure 9.3). GLP-1 is normally broken down by an enzyme called *DPP-4*. Because these drugs block the activity of the DPP-4 enzyme, they are called *DPP-4 inhibitors*. Allowing GLP-1 to stay in the body longer than usual results in the pancreas releasing more insulin but without the risk of hypoglycemia, since this hormone is only released when there is food in the gut (that is, with meals). All this results in better blood glucose levels.

How Are DPP-4 Inhibitors Taken?

These medications can be taken with or without food. The treatment plan will differ for each individual, but in general:

- Sitagliptin is taken once a day; the provider will prescribe doses of either 25, 50, or 100 mg.
- Saxagliptin is taken once a day; the provider will prescribe doses of either 2.5 or 5 mg.
- Linagliptin is taken once a day; the provider will typically prescribe a dose of 5 mg daily.
- Alogliptin is taken once a day; the provider will prescribe doses of either 6.25, 12.5, or 25 mg daily.

Facts about DPP-4 Inhibitors

- DPP-4 inhibitors are effective at lowering blood glucose levels and have a low risk of hypoglycemia.
- Dose reductions are typically needed for some of these medications in people with kidney disease. However, it should be noted that the combination pills with metformin may not be safe in those with kidney or liver disease. People generally don't gain or lose weight on these medications.
- When taken alone, DPP-4 inhibitors do not usually cause low blood glucose.

- These medications are usually well tolerated, but infrequent side effects may include nausea, diarrhea, and abdominal cramps.

Warning!
- Pregnant women should talk to their providers before taking these medications.
- There have been reports of acute pancreatitis occurring more commonly in people who use DPP-4 inhibitors, but whether this adverse effect is definitely related to the use of these medicines is unclear. If symptoms of pancreatitis develop (see "Pancreatitis" on page 149), these medications should be stopped, and the pancreatitis should be treated.

WHAT DOES IT ALL MEAN?
- DPP-4 inhibitors are a class of oral diabetes medications.
- They are commonly used in combination with other medications for diabetes.
- A benefit of this class of medicines is that they do not cause too-low blood glucose values (hypoglycemia) and are generally well tolerated.
- DPP-4 inhibitors generally lower A1C values by 0.5% to 1% (5.5 to 11 mmol/mol).

Incretin Mimetics (GLP–1 Receptor Agonists)

GLP-1 receptor agonists are injectable diabetes medications used for the treatment of type 2 diabetes. Some of the benefits of this medicine class include weight loss and minimal risk of hypoglycemia. GLP-1 receptor agonists, also known as *incretin mimetics*, are recommended for persons with type 2 diabetes who have high blood glucose levels. Most people find that their A1C levels drop, on average, by 0.5% to 1.5% (5.5 to 17 mmol/mol) on these medications.

▶ WHAT YOU NEED TO KNOW

What Are GLP-1 Receptor Agonists?
These medications are available as injections that are given under the skin. A few types of GLP-1 receptor agonists are available, such as the following:
- Dulaglutide (weekly; brand name Trulicity)
- Exenatide (twice daily; brand name Byetta)
- Exenatide extended release (weekly; brand name Bydureon)
- Liraglutide (daily; brand name Victoza)

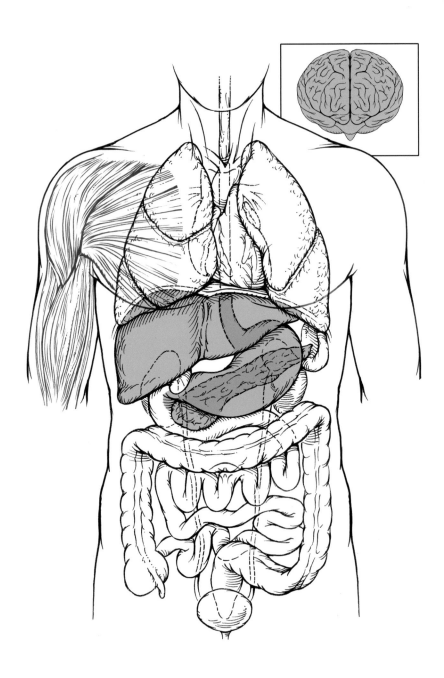

9.4 GLP-1 receptor agonists have effects on the liver (preventing glucose release), stomach (slowing food emptying), and pancreas (helping more insulin to be released when food is eaten). They may also have certain effects on areas in the brain, causing a feeling of fullness. These multiple effects result in the lowering of blood glucose levels. © 2018, Johns Hopkins University, Art as Applied to Medicine

- Lixisenatide (daily; brand name Adlyxin)
- Semaglutide (weekly; brand name Ozempic)

What Do They Do?

These medicines mimic a hormone produced by the body called GLP-1, which stimulates the pancreas to produce insulin with meals. These drugs also slow down the emptying of the stomach and keep food in the stomach longer so that people feel full sooner. They also reduce the liver's ability to break down glycogen into glucose in the blood, and they act on the brain to suppress the appetite (figure 9.4). All these effects promote healthy blood glucose levels in people with type 2 diabetes.

How Are They Taken?

The treatment plan will differ for each person, but in general:

- **Dulaglutide** People start with 0.75 mg injections weekly; after a month, the provider may increase the dose to 1.5 mg weekly.
- **Exenatide** People start with 5-microgram (mcg) injections twice daily; after a month, the health care provider may increase the dose to 10 mcg twice daily.
- **Exenatide extended release** People typically take 2 mg once weekly.
- **Liraglutide** People start with 0.6 mg once-daily injections; after a week, the health provider may increase the dose to 1.2 mg once daily. The maximum dose is 1.8 mg once daily. (Note that the 3 mg dose of this medication is marketed as Saxenda and approved as a weight-loss therapy for people with or without diabetes.)
- **Lixisenatide** People start with 10 mcg once daily; after 2 weeks the provider may increase the dose to 20 mcg daily.
- **Semaglutide** People start with 0.25 mg injections weekly and then, after 1 month, increase the dose to 0.5 mg injections weekly. After another month, the provider may increase the dose to 1 mg injections weekly.

Facts about GLP-1 Agonists

- These drugs are effective at lowering blood glucose levels and have a low risk of hypoglycemia.
- Overweight or obese people generally lose weight on these medications; on average, people lose about 6.5 pounds (3 kilograms).
- These medications must be injected.
- Some people have gastrointestinal side effects when taking these drugs, such as nausea, vomiting, diarrhea, and abdominal cramps.

- Some GLP-1 receptor agonists have been found to reduce recurrent heart attacks or stroke and premature death in people with a previous history of cardiovascular disease. Liraglutide is currently the only medication in this class approved by the Food and Drug Administration (FDA) to have a cardiovascular benefit.

Warning!
- Pregnant women should talk to their providers before taking these medications.
- GLP-1 receptor agonists have been associated with a potential increased risk for pancreatitis (see "Pancreatitis" on page 149). This risk overall is very low, but these medicines should not be used in people with a prior history of pancreatitis.

WHAT DOES IT ALL MEAN?
- GLP-1 receptor agonists are a class of injectable medications for type 2 diabetes dosed twice daily, daily, or weekly.
- Benefits include weight loss and a low risk for hypoglycemia.
- Typical side effects include gastrointestinal upset, such as nausea, vomiting, bloating, and diarrhea. These medications can slow the absorption of other pills and should not be used in people with a history of gastroparesis (see "Gastroparesis" on page 141).
- GLP-1 agonists generally lower A1C values by 0.5% to 1.5% (5.5 to 17 mmol/mol).
- There may be additional heart protection benefits for some drugs in this class among people who have a history of heart disease or stroke.

SGLT2 Inhibitors

Sodium glucose cotransporter 2 (SGLT2) inhibitors are a class of oral medicines used to treat type 2 diabetes. SGLT2 inhibitors are recommended for persons with type 2 diabetes who have high blood glucose levels. On average, these medications reduce the A1C by 0.5% to 1% (5.5 to 11 mmol/mol).

▶ WHAT YOU NEED TO KNOW

What Are SGLT2 Inhibitors?

These medications are available as an oral tablet. There are three SGLT2 inhibitors currently available:

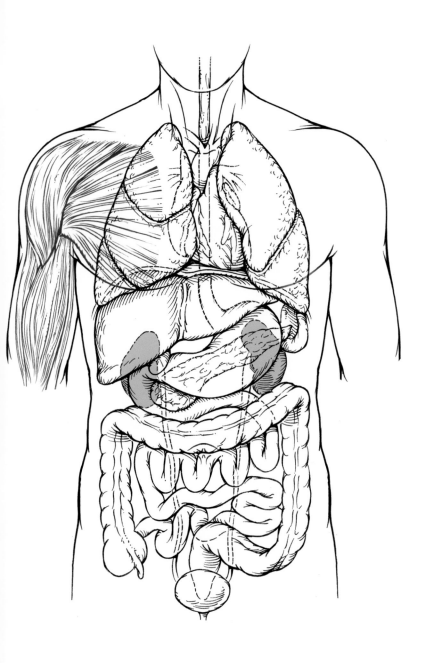

9.5 SGLT2 inhibitors act on the kidneys, preventing the reabsorption of glucose back into the body. This results in glucose leaving in the urine instead and lowering blood glucose levels. © 2018, Johns Hopkins University, Art as Applied to Medicine

- Canagliflozin (brand name Invokana)
- Dapagliflozin (brand name Farxiga)
- Empagliflozin (brand name Jardiance)

What Do They Do?

These pills work by preventing filtered glucose from being reabsorbed by the kidneys back into the bloodstream from the urine (figure 9.5). As a result, they decrease glucose levels in the blood and cause it to spill into the urine.

How Are They Taken?

The treatment plan will differ for each person, but in general SGLT2 inhibitors are taken once a day before the first meal. The typical dose is 100 to 300 mg (canagliflozin), 5 to 10 mg (dapagliflozin), or 10 to 25 mg (empagliflozin). In most cases, SGLT2 inhibitors are used in addition to other diabetes medications and are available in combination pills with metformin.

Facts about SGLT2 Inhibitors

- These drugs are effective at lowering blood glucose levels and have a low risk of hypoglycemia.
- Some people report mild weight loss after taking SGLT2 inhibitors.
- Alone, these medications are associated with a low risk of hypoglycemia.
- SGLT2 inhibitors may increase urination and raise the risk of yeast infections and urinary tract infections. These drugs can also lead to low blood pressure.
- Kidney function needs to be tested before and during treatment with SGLT2 inhibitors.
- Some SGLT2 inhibitors (empagliflozin and canagliflozin) have been found to reduce recurrent heart attacks or stroke in people with a previous history of heart disease or stroke and may delay or prevent the progression of kidney disease. Empagliflozin is currently the only medication in this class approved by the FDA to reduce premature death from cardiovascular disease.

Warning!

- Women who are pregnant or who are breastfeeding should talk to their care providers before taking these medications.
- SGLT2 inhibitors have been associated with a higher risk of diabetic ketoacidosis (DKA). In people taking SGLT2 inhibitors, DKA can present with near-normal glucose values. Any person with persistent nausea, vomiting, weakness, or abdominal pain while taking an SGLT2 inhibitor

should be evaluated for DKA even if his or her glucose values are not markedly elevated.

- Amputations are a serious but rare risk associated with the use of the SGLT2 inhibitor canagliflozin. Fractures are also more common with the use of canagliflozin.
- People with severe kidney disease should not use SGLT2 inhibitors. Though SGLT2 inhibitors have been used in people with type 1 diabetes, the safety of these drugs has not been extensively studied in this population and are not currently approved by the FDA for the management of type 1 diabetes.

WHAT DOES IT ALL MEAN?

- SGLT2 inhibitors are a class of oral medications for type 2 diabetes.
- They are commonly used in combination with other medications for diabetes.
- The benefits of this class of medicines include mild weight loss and a low risk of hypoglycemia.
- SGLT2 inhibitors generally lower A1C values by 0.5% to 1% (5.5 to 11 mmol/mol).
- There may be additional heart protection benefits for some drugs in this class among people who have a history of heart disease or stroke.

Sulfonylureas and Other Secretagogues

Sulfonylureas and meglitinides are oral medications used to treat type 2 diabetes that are collectively categorized as *insulin secretagogues*. This term simply means that these medications stimulate insulin release from the pancreas. Sulfonylureas and meglitinides are recommended for persons with type 2 diabetes who have high blood glucose levels. On average, most people find that their A1C levels drop by 1% to 1.5% (11 to 17 mmol/mol) with sulfonylureas and 0.5% to 1% (5.5 to 11 mmol/mol) with meglitinides.

▶ WHAT YOU NEED TO KNOW

What Are Sulfonylureas and Meglitinides?

These medications are available as oral tablets. Sulfonylureas stimulate the pancreas to release insulin over a period of several hours. Common brands include the following:

- Glipizide (brand name Glucotrol)
- Glyburide (brand names DiaBeta Glynase and Micronase)

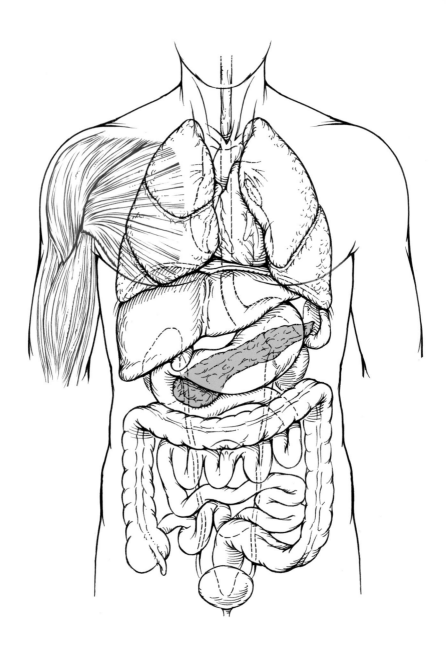

9.6 Sulfonylureas and meglitinides both act on the pancreas, causing more insulin to be released into the blood and lowering blood glucose levels. © 2018, Johns Hopkins University, Art as Applied to Medicine

- Glimepiride (brand name Amaryl)

Meglitinides stimulate a shorter-term burst of insulin to cover mealtimes and are taken multiple times per day before meals. Common brands include the following:

- Repaglinide (brand name Prandin)
- Nateglinide (brand name Starlix)

What Do They Do?

Sulfonylureas and meglitinides work by directly stimulating the hormone-releasing cells (*islets*) in the pancreas to release more insulin (figure 9.6).

How Are They Taken?

Sulfonylureas are usually taken once or twice a day, in the morning, evening, or both, depending on the medication:

- Glipizide (brand name Glucotrol) is usually taken once or twice a day; a typical daily dose is 5 mg to a maximum of 40 mg.
- Glipizide extended release (brand name Glucotrol XL) is usually taken once a day; a typical daily dose is 5 mg to a maximum of 20 mg.
- Glyburide (brand name DiaBeta, Micronase, or Glynase) is taken once or twice a day; a typical daily dose is 1.25 mg to a maximum of 20 mg.
- Glimepiride (brand name Amaryl) is taken once a day; a typical dose is 1 to 4 mg; maximum 8 mg daily.

Meglitinides are usually taken 15 to 30 minutes before each meal:

- Repaglinide (brand name Prandin) is taken at doses usually ranging from 0.5 to 4 mg with each meal.
- Nateglinide (brand name Starlix) is taken at doses usually ranging from 60 to 120 mg with each meal.

Combination pills with metformin are available.

Facts about Sulfonylureas

- Sulfonylureas are very effective at managing blood glucose levels and lowering the A1C.
- Sulfonylureas can result in hypoglycemia if the person skips a meal. This tends to occur more often in people who are older or have kidney disease and take glyburide.
- People with worsening kidney function may need to reduce their dose or stop these medications and should not take glyburide.
- People tend to gain a few pounds of weight on these medications.
- These medications tend to be less effective the longer they are used and the longer a person has had diabetes.

Warning!

- Pregnant women should exercise caution and talk to their health care providers before taking this medication. If used, glyburide is considered the safest sulfonylurea during pregnancy.
- There is a warning for a potentially increased risk of heart disease based on studies of older medications in this class that are no longer available. However, in general, these medications are thought to be safe.

WHAT DOES IT ALL MEAN?

- Sulfonylureas and meglitinides are oral medications used to treat type 2 diabetes that can be used in combination with other medications for diabetes.
- They can be effective at treating type 2 diabetes, generally lowering A1C up to 1.5% (17 mmol/mol).
- These medications, particularly glyburide, carry a risk of hypoglycemia, which can limit their use. If used in combination with insulin therapy, doses may need to be reduced.

Thiazolidinediones

Thiazolidinediones are a class of oral diabetes medicines used to treat type 2 diabetes. Thiazolidinediones are recommended for persons with type 2 diabetes who have high blood glucose levels and can lower A1C up to 1.5% (17 mmol/mol).

▶ WHAT YOU NEED TO KNOW

What Are Thiazolidinediones?

These medications are available as oral tablets. There are two thiazolidinediones that are currently available:

- Pioglitazone (brand name Actos)
- Rosiglitazone (brand name Avandia). Rosiglitazone use was restricted in 2011 over concerns that the medicine increased the risk of heart attacks. The FDA took away restrictions on the medicine in 2015 after further research did not demonstrate an increased heart attack risk.

Combination pills containing pioglitazone and rosiglitazone, along with other diabetes medications, such as metformin, are available.

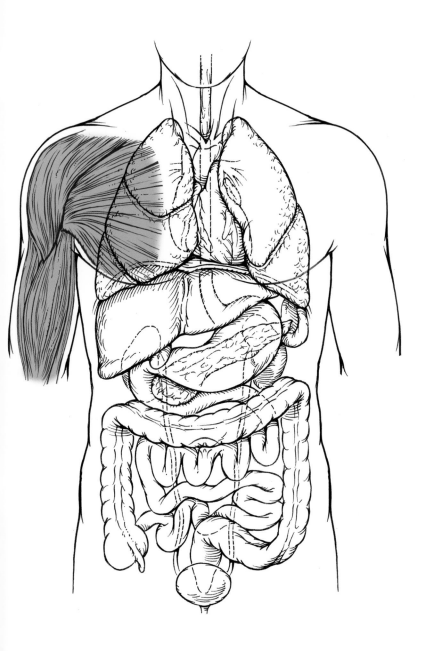

9.7 Thiazolidinediones act mainly to increase the sensitivity of skeletal muscle to insulin, thus allowing more glucose to be taken up by muscle and lowering the blood glucose levels. They may also have effects on improving the sensitivity of the liver to insulin. © 2018, Johns Hopkins University, Art as Applied to Medicine

What Do They Do?

These pills are insulin sensitizers. They reduce insulin resistance and work by enhancing the body's ability to respond to insulin, primarily in the skeletal muscle, and may improve insulin sensitivity in the liver and fat tissue as well (figure 9.7).

How Are They Taken?

The treatment plan will differ for each person, but in general:

- Pioglitazone is taken once a day; the typical dose is 15, 30, or 45 mg daily.
- Rosiglitazone is generally taken once or twice daily, starting with 2 to 4 mg once or twice daily to a maximum daily dose of 8 mg.

Facts about Thiazolidinediones

- These medications are very effective at managing blood glucose levels and lowering the A1C.
- When taken alone, these medications do not usually lead to low blood glucose levels.
- People may experience fluid retention and weight gain while taking thiazolidinedione drugs.
- People who take these drugs are more prone to bone fractures.

Warning!

- Women who are pregnant or who are breastfeeding should talk to their care providers before taking these medications.
- Studies suggest that pioglitazone may be associated with the development of bladder cancer, but the evidence is not conclusive.
- Rosiglitazone and pioglitazone may cause or worsen heart failure and are not recommended in persons with a history of heart failure.

WHAT DOES IT ALL MEAN?

- Thiazolidinediones are a class of oral medications for treating type 2 diabetes and can be used with other medications for diabetes.
- Safety concerns and side effects, such as weight gain, fluid retention, worsening heart failure, and bone fractures, have limited widespread use of these medicines.
- Thiazolidinediones generally lower A1C values by 1% to 1.5% (11 to 17 mmol/mol).

Bromocriptine

Bromocriptine is a medication that has been used for many years to treat Parkinson's disease and certain pituitary tumors. This medication can also be used to treat diabetes.

▶ WHAT YOU NEED TO KNOW

What Is Bromocriptine?

Bromocriptine is a medication that can also be used to treat people with poorly controlled type 2 diabetes. This drug can help keep blood glucose levels in a healthy range when taken as part of a healthy lifestyle.

What Does It Do?

It is a medication that mimics the neurotransmitter dopamine in the brain by activating dopamine receptors (figure 9.8). Though the exact mechanism isn't clear, this results in an improvement of blood glucose levels.

How Is It Taken?

This medication is available as an oral tablet. It works best when taken within 2 hours of waking up and when taken with food.

- Cycloset (brand name) is a tablet taken by mouth that should be initiated at one tablet (0.8 mg) and increased by one tablet per week until a maximum daily dose of six tablets (4.8 mg) or until the maximal tolerated number of tablets, between two and six per day, is reached.

Facts about Bromocriptine

- Most of the time, bromocriptine is not a first-line agent, as it decreases A1C by 0.5% to 1% (5.5 to 11 mmol/mol). Instead, it is usually taken with other diabetes medications.
- Most people start by taking a small dose, such as 0.8 mg daily, and gradually increase to a final target dose determined by their health care provider.
- Common side effects include nausea, vomiting, headache, sinus drainage, constipation, diarrhea, loss of appetite, or general stomach upset.
- Initially, bromocriptine may cause drowsiness or brief dizziness when standing after sitting or lying down for long periods. These side effects may go away once your body adjusts to the new medication.
- In rare cases, hallucinations may occur, so this may not be a good medication for those with mental illness.

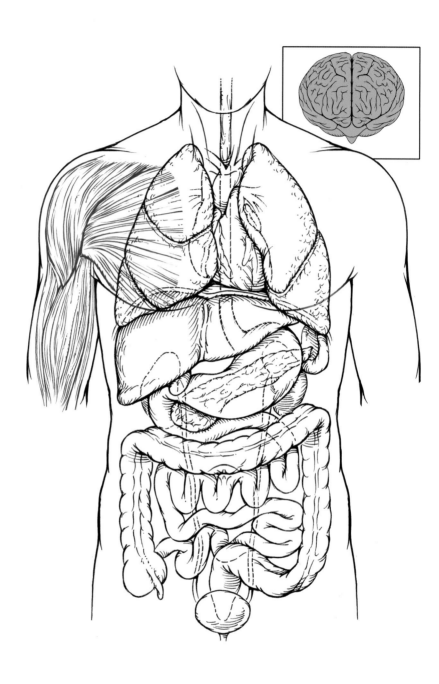

9.8 Bromocriptine stimulates dopamine receptors in the brain. Through mechanisms that remain unclear, this results in the lowering of blood glucose levels.
© 2018, Johns Hopkins University, Art as Applied to Medicine

- Although approved for the treatment of type 2 diabetes, bromocriptine is less commonly prescribed.

Warning!
- This medication should not be taken by people with severe psychotic disorders, as it may worsen compulsive behavior.
- Before taking this medication, tell your provider if you suffer from migraine headaches that involve fainting.
- In rare cases, some people have reported experiencing hallucinations when taking this medication. Tell your provider if this happens.
- Talk to your provider if you are pregnant before taking this medication.
- This medication is not recommended to be taken with some CYP3A4 inhibitors (such as HIV medications).

WHAT DOES IT ALL MEAN?
- Bromocriptine was initially developed as a medication for Parkinson's disease and certain pituitary tumors.
- Bromocriptine can be used to treat diabetes as well, typically in combination with other medications.
- Dizziness and drowsiness may occur when first starting bromocriptine, so be cautious.
- The A1C-lowering effect is 0.5% to 1% (5.5 to 11 mmol/mol).

Amylin Analogs

Amylin is a hormone that helps control glucose levels. Like insulin, amylin is made by beta cells in the pancreas and released into the bloodstream when a person begins to eat. People with type 1 diabetes make no amylin, while amylin is produced in lower amounts in those having type 2 diabetes.

▶ WHAT YOU NEED TO KNOW

What Is Pramlintide?
Pramlintide is an amylin analog, a drug form of amylin that is injected under the skin before meals. It can be used in people with type 1 diabetes and in people with type 2 diabetes who use mealtime insulin.

What Does It Do?
Amylin analogs decrease the release of glucagon, a hormone that causes the

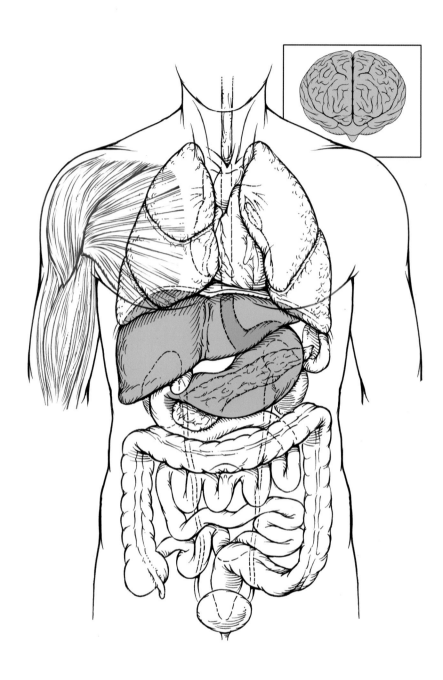

9.9 Amylin analogs slow food leaving the stomach, act on the brain to make you feel full, and prevent the liver from releasing glucose into the blood. © 2018, Johns Hopkins University, Art as Applied to Medicine

liver to release too much glucose in people with diabetes. Amylin analogs also slow how fast the stomach empties after a meal and help control the appetite (figure 9.9). These actions lower after-meal glucose levels and often lead to a small weight loss.

How Is It Taken?

When starting pramlintide in people with type 1 diabetes, mealtime insulin doses need to be reduced to prevent hypoglycemia.

- Pramlintide (brand name Symlin) is an injectable medication taken before meals that is available in a pen formulation.
- For people with type 2 diabetes, the starting dose is 60 mcg injected immediately prior to each major meal. The dose may be increased from 60 to 120 mcg before each major meal when no significant nausea has occurred for at least 3 days.
- For people with type 1 diabetes, pramlintide is started at 15 mcg and injected immediately prior to each major meal. The dose may be increased in 15 mcg increments (to doses of 30, 45, or 60 mcg) when no significant nausea has occurred for at least 3 days.
- If significant nausea persists, the dose of pramlintide may need to be decreased.

Facts about Pramlintide

- Most of the time, pramlintide is not a first-line agent, as it decreases A1C by 0.5% to 1% (5.5 to 11 mmol/mol). Instead, it is usually taken with other diabetes medications. In fact, it is only approved for use in persons with diabetes who are already taking mealtime insulin.
- Pramlintide decreases insulin requirements and leads to a weight loss of about 1 to 2 pounds, on average, in persons with type 1 diabetes. In persons with type 2 diabetes, body weight tends not to change with pramlintide use.
- The most common side effect of pramlintide is nausea, the likelihood of which can be lowered by starting a low dose and gradually increasing to higher doses.
- The amount of pramlintide you use will depend on whether you have type 1 or type 2 diabetes.
- Pramlintide and insulin should always be administered as separate injections and never mixed.

Warning!
- Talk to your provider if you are pregnant before taking this medication.

Colesevelam
(see "Bile Acid Sequestrants" on page 284)

TYPES OF INSULIN
Basal (Intermediate- and Long-Acting) Insulins

Basal (intermediate- and long-acting) insulins have a long-lasting effect throughout the day. Basal insulins are recommended for people with type 1, type 2, or gestational diabetes. They may also be used in other types of diabetes (for example, steroid-induced).

Persons with type 1 diabetes use intermediate-acting insulin or long-acting insulin in conjunction with regular or rapid-acting insulin. Persons with type 2 diabetes may use intermediate- or long-acting insulins alone or in conjunction with regular or rapid-acting insulins or with oral medications. Non-insulin injectable therapy (that is, GLP-1 agonists) can also be used with insulin. There is theoretically no maximum A1C-lowering effect for insulin therapy.

▶ WHAT YOU NEED TO KNOW
What Are Basal Insulins?

These medications are given as injections under the skin and are not suitable for insulin pumps.

The most common type of intermediate-acting insulin:

- NPH (brand names Humulin N or Novolin N; available in vials or pens)

Long-acting insulins are marketed as different brands. The common ones:
- Glargine (brand names Lantus, Basaglar, and Toujeo. Lantus is available in vials and pens. Basaglar and Toujeo are only available as pens.) Toujeo

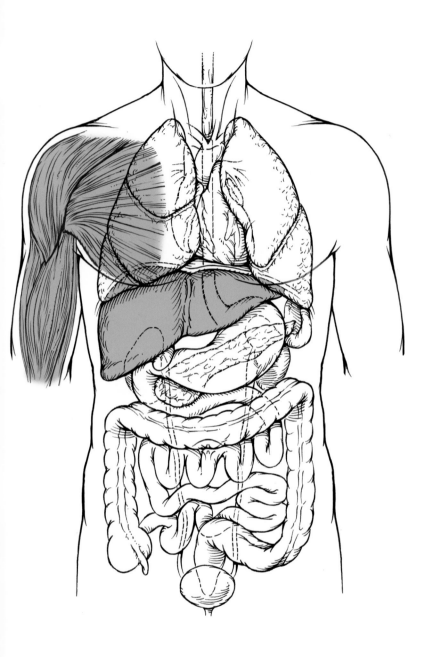

9.10 Insulin acts directly on the muscles and fat, stimulating these organs to take up glucose from the blood and use it as an energy source or store it for future needs. It also prevents the breakdown of glucose stores (*glycogen*) in the liver from entering the bloodstream. © 2018, Johns Hopkins University, Art as Applied to Medicine

(U-300) is three times more concentrated than other forms of glargine (known as U-100 insulin).
- Detemir (brand name Levemir and available in vials and pens).
- Degludec (brand name Tresiba and only available as pens). Insulin degludec comes in the usual concentration (U-100) but also comes in a version that is two times more concentrated (U-200).

What Do They Do?

These medicines are injected into the tissue under the skin and are slowly released into the body. These insulins allow glucose from the bloodstream to enter the cells in the body (primarily in muscle and fat tissue) so that it can be used as energy and potentially stored for future use. It also prevents the glycogen in the liver from breaking down and entering as glucose into the bloodstream (figure 9.10).

How Are They Taken, and How Long Are They Effective?

- NPH insulin is usually injected once or twice a day. It begins working 1 to 3 hours after injection and is most effective between 4 and 10 hours of injection. It generally keeps working for 10 to 16 hours.
- Insulin detemir can be used once or twice a day. It begins working a few hours after injection and generally keeps working anywhere from 20 to 24 hours.
- Insulin glargine is usually injected once a day. It begins working a few hours after injection and remains effective until it wears off 24 hours later. The more concentrated version of insulin glargine (Toujeo) can remain effective longer.
- Insulin degludec is injected once a day. It begins working a few hours after injection and is the most long-acting insulin, with effects that are longer than 24 hours.
- Basal insulins can be injected with a traditional syringe and needle (figure 9.12) or with a disposable pen that has been prefilled with insulin (figure 9.13). Pens, while convenient, can be more expensive.

Facts about Basal Insulins

- When NPH and regular insulin are injected together, people should first draw up the clear regular insulin, followed by the cloudy NPH insulin. Always remember: clear first, cloudy second. Never mix detemir, glargine, or degludec with other insulins.

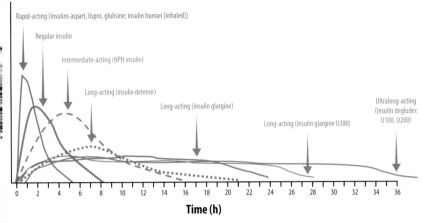

Rapid-acting (insulins aspart, lispro, glulisine; insulin human [inhaled])

Regular insulin

Intermediate-acting (NPH insulin)

Long-acting (insulin detemir)

Long-acting (insulin glargine)

Long-acting (insulin glargine U300)

Ultralong-acting (insulin degludec U100, U200)

Time (h)

9.11 Each intermediate- and long-acting insulin has a different time to reach its peak effectiveness and duration of effect. © 2018, Johns Hopkins University, Art as Applied to Medicine

- People with kidney or liver problems can take these insulins, but reduced doses may be needed.
- Insulin that is kept warm, rather than at room temperature, may be absorbed too quickly by the body and result in too-low blood glucose levels. Massaging the site of injection also speeds the absorption of insulin, as can exercise.
- Intermediate- and long-acting insulins should not be used in pumps.
- These insulins may sometimes but not always require dose reductions if you are fasting prior to a procedure.
- People with type 1 diabetes always need to take their basal insulin daily.
- Some people have hardening of the fat tissue, which appears as soft lumps of fat (*lipohypertrophy*), loss of fat tissue below the skin (*lipoatrophy*), or scarring of fat tissue (*lipodystrophy*) at the site of insulin injections. This can be avoided by rotating to a different insulin injection site every few days and always using a new syringe or pen needle with each injection. For instance, if injecting in the abdomen, rotate injections with each injection at least 1 inch (or two finger widths) apart from the time before.

Warning!
- Pregnant women are sometimes prescribed the human insulin NPH because it is the most widely studied basal insulin for pregnancy. The other

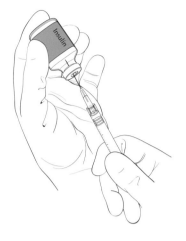

9.12 When using insulin from a vial, a syringe is used to draw it up and inject it. © 2018, Johns Hopkins University, Art as Applied to Medicine

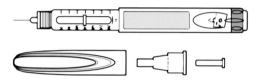

9.13 When using a pen prefilled with insulin, a dose is usually chosen by rotating the dial, and then insulin is injected through a needle attached to the pen. © 2018, Johns Hopkins University, Art as Applied to Medicine

basal insulins (such as detemir) may also be safe, but talk to your health care provider before taking any of the basal insulins during pregnancy.

WHAT DOES IT ALL MEAN?

- Basal insulins are intermediate- and long-acting insulins used for the treatment of type 1 diabetes and for some people with type 2 diabetes.
- Like all types of insulins, the basal insulins have a side effect of hypoglycemia.

Bolus (Short- and Rapid-Acting) Insulins

Bolus insulins are short-acting (regular) and rapid-acting (aspart, lispro, glulisine) insulins that can be used to treat people with type 1 and type 2 diabetes. They may also be used in other types of diabetes. These medications can be used together with basal insulins, non-insulin injectable therapies, and oral medications for diabetes.

There is theoretically no maximum A1C-lowering effect for insulin therapy.

► WHAT YOU NEED TO KNOW

What Are Bolus Insulins?

These medications are given as injections under the skin. Most are also suitable for use in insulin pumps.

Rapid-acting insulins can be injected with a traditional syringe and needle or with a disposable pen. Pens, though convenient, may be expensive. There are three common rapid-acting insulins:

- Aspart (brand name NovoLog, NovoLog FlexPen, Fiasp, Fiasp FlexTouch pen)
- Lispro (brand name Humalog, Humalog KwikPen, Admelog, Admelog SoloSTAR pen)
- Glulisine (brand name Apidra and the Apidra SoloSTAR pen)

Regular insulin is marketed by a few different companies:

- Regular insulin (brand names Novolin R or Humulin R)

What Do They Do?

These medicines are injected into the soft tissues under the skin. They act quickly and for a short period of time to help the body utilize carbohydrates from meals. These insulins allow glucose from the bloodstream to enter cells, primarily in the skeletal muscle or fat tissue, so that glucose can be used as energy or stored for future use. Insulin also prevents the liver from breaking down glycogen and releasing glucose into the bloodstream (figure 9.10).

How Are They Taken, and How Long
Are They Effective?

Rapid-acting insulins are injected within 15 minutes of eating or immediately afterward. They are most effective 1 to 2 hours after injection and stop working in approximately 4 hours.

Regular insulin is not absorbed as quickly, so it is usually injected 30 minutes before each meal. It begins working in 30 minutes to 1 hour and is most effective 2 to 3 hours after injection. The effect wears off after 6 to 8 hours.

Facts about Bolus Insulins

- Rapid-acting insulins are often used in insulin pumps.
- Rapid-acting insulins are newer than regular insulin and act with a faster onset but are more expensive.
- Bolus insulins can be injected with a traditional syringe and needle (figure 9.12) or with a disposable pen that has been prefilled with insulin (figure 9.13). Pens, while convenient, can be more expensive.

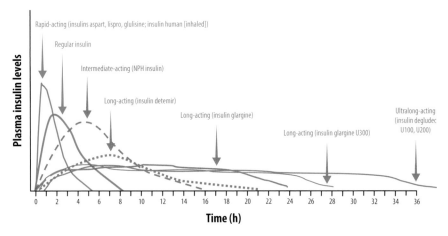

Plasma insulin levels

Rapid-acting (insulins aspart, lispro, glulisine; insulin human [inhaled])

Regular insulin

Intermediate-acting (NPH insulin)

Long-acting (insulin detemir)

Long-acting (insulin glargine)

Long-acting (insulin glargine U300)

Ultralong-acting (insulin degludec U100, U200)

Time (h)

9.14 Rapid-acting insulins and regular insulin each have a different time to reach their peak effectiveness and duration of effect. © 2018, Johns Hopkins University, Art as Applied to Medicine

- These insulins can result in hypoglycemia if they are injected before a meal and the person delays eating or eats less than expected. Hypoglycemia can also result if too much insulin is injected in a short period of time. Always give the medication time to work before injecting any additional insulin.

- Combining regular insulin or rapid-acting insulin with oral medicines to treat type 2 diabetes may increase the risk of low blood glucose (particularly with sulfonylureas). Doses of oral and other non-insulin injectable medicines for diabetes may need to be adjusted when adding insulin.

- Some people have a hardening of fat tissue that appears as soft lumps of fat, loss of fat tissue below the skin, or scarring of fat tissue at the site of insulin injections. This can be avoided by rotating to a different insulin injection site every few days and always using a new syringe or pen needle with each injection. For instance, if injecting in the abdomen, rotate injections with each injection at least 1 inch (or two finger widths) apart from the time before.

Warning!
- Aspart, lispro, and regular insulin are generally safe to use during pregnancy, but always check with your provider first when using any of the bolus insulins.

- Bolus insulins are short- or rapid-acting insulins that are used for the treatment of diabetes.
- These insulins are generally given just before a meal to help manage blood glucose spikes from ingested carbohydrates. They can also be used to "correct" or lower very high blood glucose values.
- More concentrated versions of some bolus insulins are also available.
- Like all types of insulins, bolus insulins have a risk of causing hypoglycemia, especially if food intake is reduced or delayed or if physical activity is increased. Self-monitoring of blood glucose levels is important for people taking insulin therapy.

Inhaled Insulin

Inhaled insulin is a rapid-acting insulin that is delivered by an inhaler. This drug is approved for people with type 1 and 2 diabetes who have poorly managed blood glucose levels as an alternative to injectable rapid-acting insulin.

▶ WHAT YOU NEED TO KNOW

What Is Inhaled Insulin?

Inhaled insulin (brand name Afrezza) is different from other insulins because it is inhaled instead of injected. Inhaled insulin works more quickly than insulin that's injected because it enters the bloodstream more quickly.

What Does It Do?

Like other forms of insulin, inhaled insulin works on the liver, muscle, and fat tissues to take up glucose to be used as an energy source and blocks the liver from releasing glucose into the bloodstream (figure 9.10).

How Is It Taken?

The treatment plan will differ for each individual, but most people take an initial dose of four units of Afrezza at the beginning of each meal. People who are already taking mealtime insulin may require a different dose, as described in table 9.1.

Facts about Inhaled Insulin

- Before starting this medication, your provider should perform a thorough exam to determine if you have any signs of lung disease.
- This medication may cause mild weight gain, like all insulin.
- Hypoglycemia is a possible side effect, similar to other insulins.

Table 9.1. Converting injectable bolus insulin to inhaled insulin units

INJECTABLE INSULIN (REGULAR, HUMALOG, NOVOLOG, APIDRA)	INHALED INSULIN (AFREZZA)
up to 4 units	4 units
5–8 units	8 units
9–12 units	12 units
13–16 units	16 units
17–20 units	20 units
21–24 units	24 units

Warning!
- Breathing tests that assess lung function (for example, spirometry) are needed before and after starting this drug, since small declines in lung function can occur while using this medication.
- Inhaled insulin may cause a sore throat and occasional breathing problems due to spasm of the upper airways, even in people whose lungs were healthy when they began taking the medication. Rare cases of lung cancer have been reported in users of inhaled insulin, but it's not clear whether the inhaled insulin contributed to the cancer in any way.
- Inhaled insulin is not recommended for people who smoke or recently stopped smoking or for persons with asthma, chronic obstructive pulmonary disease (COPD), or active lung cancer.
- Inhaled insulin must be used along with long-acting insulin in people with type 1 diabetes.
- Inhaled insulin is not recommended for the treatment of diabetic ketoacidosis.

WHAT DOES IT ALL MEAN?
- Inhaled insulin is a rapid-acting insulin taken before meals as an alternative to injected rapid-acting insulin.

- For those being switched to inhaled insulin, guidelines are available that recommend the dose of Afrezza to use based on the dose of the premeal injected insulin used.
- The dose ranges of inhaled insulin may be more limited. Inhaled insulin can cause airways to spasm and therefore should not be used in persons who smoke or in those who have asthma or COPD.
- Inhaled insulin usage requires that lung function tests be measured before starting therapy and periodically thereafter. This insulin results in predictable reductions in lung function over time.

Premixed Insulin Preparations

Premixed insulin, as the name implies, is when two different insulins having different actions are combined. Usually, this includes a basal insulin and a bolus insulin mixed together in one injection. This therapy is an option for people with type 1, type 2, or gestational diabetes who need to give multiple daily insulin shots and reduces the total number of insulin injections per day.

▶ WHAT YOU NEED TO KNOW

What Are Premixed Insulins?

Premixed insulin has two components:

- Short-acting (regular) insulin or rapid-acting (lispro, aspart, and glulisine) insulin (bolus insulins)
  - Needed at meals to help the body lower blood glucose levels after eating
- Intermediate-acting insulin (basal insulins)
  - Needed throughout the day to regulate blood glucose levels between meals
  - Available in two forms:
    - Neutral protamine Hagedorn (NPH)
    - Insulin analogs, such as insulin aspart protamine or insulin lispro protamine, are man-made. Note the *protamine* part of the name, which distinguishes these from their rapid-acting relatives.

What Do They Do?

The premixed insulins work similarly to the basal and bolus insulins (figure 9.10). The only difference is that they are mixed together in one injection in a fixed-dose combination.

Table 9.2. Insulin components of common premixed insulin preparations

RATIO	CONTENTS	GENERIC NAME	BRAND NAME
70/30	Intermediate insulin (70%) Short- or rapid-acting insulin (30%)	70% human insulin isophane suspension and 30% human insulin injection (*premix NPH/regular insulin 70/30*)	Novolin 70/30, Humulin 70/30
		70% insulin aspart protamine suspension and 30% insulin aspart injection (*premix insulin aspart 70/30*)	Novolog Mix 70/30
75/25	Intermediate insulin (75%) Rapid-acting insulin (25%)	75% insulin lispro protamine suspension and 25% insulin lispro injection (*premix insulin lispro 75/25*)	Humalog Mix 75/25
50/50	Intermediate insulin (50%) Rapid-acting insulin (50%)	50% insulin lispro protamine suspension and 50% insulin lispro injection (*premix insulin lispro 50/50*)	Humalog Mix 50/50

How Is It Taken?

Premixed insulin is available in three ratios (table 9.2). In these ratios the dose of intermediate-acting insulin is listed first and the rapid-acting insulin second. The ratio chosen will depend on the size of the meals a person eats from day to day. For instance, someone who eats a smaller breakfast and dinner may be started on 75/25 insulin, and someone who eats larger meals may be started on 50/50 insulin. Also, the ratio of insulin may be determined by how a person's glucose levels respond to different types of insulin.

Most people will start with a single injection every day, given within 15 to 30 minutes before the day's biggest meal.

If needed, the dose may increase to two injections per day. In some cases, premixed insulins may be given up to three times a day.

Facts about Premixed Insulins

- These products are very convenient—they reduce the number of injections, eliminate the need for calculations, and are less costly. However, they might not lower blood glucose levels as well as regimens using more injections if the person does not follow a predictable meal schedule.
- Premixed insulin is not for everyone. Certain people shouldn't use premixed insulin because of a greater risk of very high or low glucose levels. This includes persons who
    - skip meals,
    - eat meals at different times each day,
    - eat meals that are very different in size from day to day, or
    - have an unpredictable exercise schedule.
- Some people have a hardening of fat tissue that appears as soft lumps of fat, loss of fat tissue below the skin, or scarring of fat tissue at the site of insulin injections. This can be avoided by rotating to a different insulin injection site every few days and always using a new syringe or pen needle with each injection. For instance, if injecting in the abdomen, rotate injections with each injection at least 1 inch (or two finger widths) apart from the time before.

Warning!

- Lower doses may be needed in people with kidney disease because insulin may not be cleared by the kidneys as quickly.
- Lower doses may be needed in people with liver disease because insulin may not be broken down as well and may prevent the diseased liver from releasing enough glucose into the bloodstream.
- One premixed insulin product is commonly used for treating gestational diabetes: NPH/regular (brand names Novolin 70/30 and Humulin 70/30). Talk to your health care provider before taking any of the premixed insulins during pregnancy.

WHAT DOES IT ALL MEAN?

- In people with diabetes who need to be treated with multiple daily insulin shots, premixed insulins provide both short- (or rapid) and intermediate-acting insulins in one injection and decrease the number of total daily insulin injections.

- While this may be more convenient (and less costly in some cases), many people are not good candidates for premixed insulins, and diabetes management may not be as good or as safe with their use, particularly in people with unpredictable eating schedules.

U–500 Regular Concentrated Insulin

U-500 insulin is a very concentrated form of regular insulin used to treat people with type 2 diabetes who are severely *insulin resistant*, meaning their bodies cannot respond to insulin appropriately. These people need high doses of insulin (often greater than 200 units) to keep their blood glucose levels in the goal range and may benefit from taking U-500 insulin to reduce the volume of medication injected.

▶ WHAT YOU NEED TO KNOW

What Is U-500 Insulin?

- Regular insulin U-500 (brand name Humulin R U-500) is injected using a special U-500 insulin syringe under the skin multiple times per day.
- It is also available as an insulin pen.

What Does It Do?

Insulin helps transport glucose into the cells of the body (fat and muscle) to be used as energy and prevents glycogen in the liver from breaking down into glucose and entering the bloodstream (figure 9.10). Some people with diabetes need to take U-500 insulin because their body does not respond effectively enough to the insulin it produces and is tremendously insulin resistant.

How Is It Taken?

U-500 regular insulin can be injected several times a day, depending on your body's needs.

- U-500 insulin is five times more concentrated than the standard form of insulin, known as U-100 insulin. People with diabetes can take very small volumes (one-fifth) of U-500 to achieve the same results they might get from a large dose of U-100.
- To avoid an accidental overdose, do not use a standard insulin syringe to inject U-500. Use a special syringe, made specifically for U-500, that takes into account these important differences in drug concentrations, or use the U-500 insulin pen.
- The U-500 insulin pen does not require dose conversions.

Facts about U-500 Insulin

- Like other forms of insulin, side effects include accidental drops in blood glucose, weight gain, redness, and pain or itching at the injection site.
- Taking U-500 along with other drugs that lower blood glucose can increase the risk of hypoglycemia.
- Because it is highly concentrated, the duration of action for U-500 insulin is similar to that of basal or intermediate-acting insulins. For this reason, it is usually dosed two to four times a day and prescribed as the sole insulin; all other insulins are discontinued.

Warning!

- Pregnant women should talk to their providers before taking this medication.
- Dangerous drops in blood sugar could occur if an overdose occurs—even with small injections, since this type of insulin is five times more concentrated than standard U-100 insulin. Always use a special U-500 insulin syringe before using U-500 insulin.
- Some people have a hardening of the fat tissue that appears as soft lumps of fat, loss of fat tissue below the skin, or scarring of fat tissue at the site of insulin injections. This can be avoided by rotating to a different insulin injection site every few days and always using a new syringe or pen needle with each injection. For instance, if injecting in the abdomen, rotate injections with each injection at least 1 inch (or two finger widths) apart from the time before.

WHAT DOES IT ALL MEAN?

- U-500 insulin is five times more concentrated than standard U-100 insulin, meaning there is five times more insulin per set volume.
- U-500 insulin is prescribed to some persons with diabetes who are extremely insulin resistant to help reduce the otherwise high volumes of medication they might need.

COMPLEMENTARY AND ALTERNATIVE TREATMENTS FOR DIABETES

Complementary and Alternative Medicines

Complementary and alternative treatments refer to therapies that fall outside the realm of Western conventional medicine. While these approaches generally have less scientific data supporting them, they still may have utility in treating certain conditions by themselves or along with mainstream Western approaches.

► WHAT YOU NEED TO KNOW

While complementary and alternative therapies for diabetes are quite common and in some cases have been used for hundreds of years, very little is known about how they work and whether they help, or hinder, the treatment of diabetes.

The FDA, which ensures marketed drugs are safe to use, does not test herbs, supplements, or vitamins for effectiveness or safety. In some cases, people have experienced dangerous drug interactions between alternative remedies and other drugs.

For that reason, it is important to tell your health care provider about any supplements or herbal remedies you use and only buy them from a trusted source. A few common alternative and complementary medicines are listed here; there may be others.

Complementary and Alternative Medicines for Diabetes

Bitter Melon

Bitter melon, a plant in the squash family, is a traditional remedy used in many cultures to enhance the body's response to insulin. Some trials have shown small benefits from bitter melon supplements, but these effects have not been observed in other trials. Bitter melon has not been shown to interact with other medications. However, its side effects include severe vomiting and diarrhea. It is not considered safe for children or pregnant women.

Vitamin D

Vitamin D is found in most daily multivitamins. A few studies have suggested that vitamin D might improve glucose levels in type 2 diabetes, but larger clinical trials have not been conclusive. The good news is that supplements containing moderate doses of vitamin D have been shown to improve bone health without interacting with other drugs or causing unwanted side effects (see "Testing for Vitamin D Deficiency" on page 185).

Chromium

Chromium is a trace element that may help the body break down carbohydrates and fats. A few small studies have found that people who lack normal amounts of chromium can lower their A1C levels by up to 0.5% (5.5 mmol/mol) if they take 200 to 1000 grams of chromium for as long as 6 months. Larger studies are needed to confirm this effect, especially in those with normal chromium levels before starting therapy. Chromium isn't yet known to interact with other medications, and no harmful side effects have been noted when used at reasonable doses.

Cinnamon

Some studies have suggested that daily supplements containing up to 6 grams of cinnamon (much more than someone might consume in her or his diet) improve blood glucose levels, but other studies have found no effects. The spice is not known to interact with other medications, and few side effects have been reported. Cinnamon is generally not recommended for pregnant women.

Fenugreek

Fenugreek is a traditional plant used in Asian and Mediterranean cultures. Though only a few studies have been conducted on this plant, some have suggested that sprinkling 10 to 100 grams of powdered fenugreek seed on meals may boost the amount of insulin made by the body. Fenugreek is not known to interact with other drugs, but it can cause uncomfortable side effects, including diarrhea, gas, and dizziness.

Ginseng

Ginseng is one of the most commonly used herbs. Ginseng has not been shown to have definite effects on glucose levels in clinical studies, but those with diabetes may take it for other reasons. Side effects include nausea, high blood pressure, headache, difficulty sleeping, and nervousness. Ginseng also interacts with a number of drugs, including the blood thinner warfarin (brand name Coumadin). Because of its side effects and drug interactions, ginseng is not generally recommended for people with diabetes.

Gymnema

Gymnema, an herb that grows in India and Sri Lanka, is known in Hindi as *gurmar*, which means "sugar destroyer." Though scientists are unsure how this herb works in the body, a few small clinical trials suggest that gymnema may improve A1C levels. Larger trials are still needed. The herb has no known side effects or drug interactions.

Vanadium

Vanadium is a trace element that affects how the body responds to insulin. Small scientific studies have suggested that daily doses of 50 to 300 mg of vanadium for 6 weeks might modestly improve A1C levels, but more studies are needed to verify these findings. Vanadium can cause uncomfortable side effects, such as bloating, nausea, and stomachaches.

- Alternative, complementary, and integrative medical approaches fall outside of Western medical practices but may be used by people to help treat diabetes.
- Some minerals and herbs have shown a small benefit on glucose levels in small studies, but larger and more rigorously conducted trials are needed to assess effectiveness and safety.
- Always be sure to tell your provider about any supplements you are taking to be sure they are monitored for interactions.

Meditation and Stress Reduction

Meditation can be an effective way to relieve stress. Stress relief, whether from meditative or other activities, can improve glycemic control and overall health.

▶ WHAT YOU NEED TO KNOW

People with diabetes often carry a heavy load when it comes to stress, anxiety, and depression. Stress takes a physical and emotional toll on the body.

Meditation is a process of spending time in quiet contemplation and can help lower stress.

Regular meditation for a few months has been scientifically shown to

- enhance mood,
- reduce anxiety and depression,
- alleviate pain,
- improve blood glucose levels (though not all trials show this), and
- reduce blood pressure.

Most scientific research has focused on the mediation programs listed here.

Transcendental Meditation

Transcendental meditation involves sitting quietly and allowing the mind to settle for as little as 20 minutes, once a day. This form of meditation is the most common in the Western world and involves a *mantra*, which is a word or phrase that a person repeats in his or her mind to help focus. A large body of research suggests this simple form of meditation can help lift depression, relieve stress, and reduce both blood pressure and blood glucose levels as part of an overall healthy lifestyle.

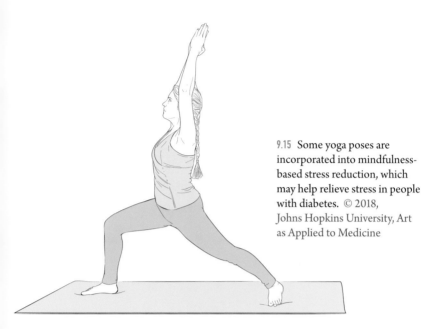

9.15 Some yoga poses are incorporated into mindfulness-based stress reduction, which may help relieve stress in people with diabetes. © 2018, Johns Hopkins University, Art as Applied to Medicine

Mindfulness-Based Programs

Mindfulness-based stress reduction (MBSR) merges body awareness and yoga with a concept called *mindfulness*. Mindfulness involves paying attention in a particular way: on purpose, in the present moment, and nonjudgmentally. By developing an awareness of how your life and the management of your diabetes interact, you can learn to respond thoughtfully, rather than just react, when challenging situations arise. The MBSR program is an 8-week workshop taught by certified trainers that includes weekly group meetings (2-hour classes), a 1-day retreat, and instruction in three formal techniques: mindfulness meditation, body scanning, and simple yoga postures (figure 9.15).

A related practice known as *mindfulness-based cognitive therapy* is helpful for people prone to anxiety, stress, and depression. People who practice this method learn to recognize the subtle thought patterns that lead to depression and relate to them in a new way to gain greater control over their mental health.

Both practices have been shown to improve stress, depressive symptoms, anxiety, and quality of life after 8 weeks of regular meditation.

Vipassana

Vipassana, an ancient form of meditation, involves sitting quietly and being mindful of breathing and the thoughts, feelings, and images that pass through your mind. This method is typically taught at a multiday (usually 10 days) silent retreat. Most mindfulness-based programs are based on Vipassana.

To engage in these activities properly, some basic training is useful. These meditation techniques are often taught by community groups, by private organizations, or through schools.

WHAT DOES IT ALL MEAN?

- Stress levels tend to be higher in those with chronic diseases, such as diabetes, and can affect the ability to self-manage diabetes at home.
- Meditation and mindfulness techniques can be helpful in reducing anxiety, depression, and stress.
- Overall stress reduction may improve glucose levels and other health problems related to diabetes.

Chapter 10

MEDICATIONS FOR CONDITIONS RELATED TO CARDIOVASCULAR DISEASE

MEDICATIONS FOR HIGH BLOOD PRESSURE
Angiotensin–Converting Enzyme Inhibitors

Angiotensin-converting enzyme (ACE) inhibitors are oral blood pressure medications. ACE inhibitors or angiotensin-receptor blockers (ARBs) are the preferred treatment for people with diabetes who have high blood pressure (*hypertension*) and the early stages of diabetic kidney disease as reflected by an elevated urine protein level (*albuminuria*). Some of these medications are also approved to treat heart failure in people with diabetes or after a myocardial infarction (heart attack) (figure 10.1).

▶ WHAT YOU NEED TO KNOW
   What Are ACE Inhibitors?
These medications are available as oral tablets. ACE inhibitors are older drugs with generic forms that are commonly prescribed. These are the most common ACE inhibitors:

- Benazepril (brand name Lotensin)
- Captopril (brand name Capoten)
- Enalapril (common brand names include Vasotec, Epaned)
- Fosinopril (brand name Monopril)
- Lisinopril (common brand names include Prinivil, Zestril)
- Ramipril (brand name Altace)

   What Do They Do?
Angiotensin II is a hormone that constricts blood vessels and leads to salt and

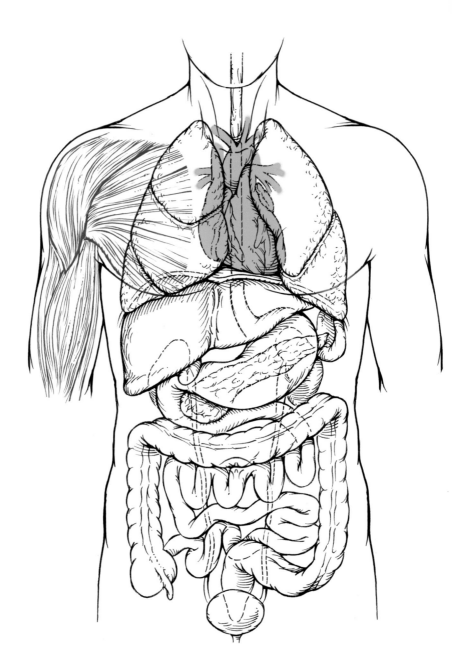

10.1 There are many medications that can be used to lower blood pressure and cholesterol and protect the heart.

© 2018, Johns Hopkins University, Art as Applied to Medicine

fluid retention in the body. This results in higher blood pressure. ACE inhibitors prevent angiotensin II from forming, hence reducing blood pressure.

How Are They Taken?

Each ACE inhibitor is given at a different dose and frequency. The dose and frequency will differ for each person; consult your health care provider for more information.

Facts about ACE Inhibitors

- ACE inhibitors are effective at controlling blood pressure.
- ACE inhibitors may be less expensive—but work just as well—as other blood pressure medications.
- In general, ACE inhibitors can slow the progression of kidney disease in people with type 1 or type 2 diabetes who have protein in their urine (see "Testing for Albuminuria" on page 156) and for this reason are preferred over other blood pressure medications for people with early kidney disease.
- Persons starting ACE inhibitors need to have blood tests to check their kidney function and potassium levels.
- Some people (5% to 20%) who take ACE inhibitors will develop a persistent, dry cough. If you experience this side effect, ask your health care provider about switching to a different class of medications (usually, an angiotensin-receptor blocker or ARB; see next topic).
- In rare cases, ACE inhibitors can cause a life-threatening condition known as *angioedema*, with severe swelling of the face, lips, and throat. If this occurs, you should go to an emergency room or call an ambulance.

Warning!

- ACE inhibitors should not be taken together with ARBs because of the risk of low blood pressure, high potassium levels, or kidney problems when combined.
- Pregnant women should *not* take ACE inhibitors. These medications have been shown to harm the unborn baby. Talk to your medical care provider about alternative blood pressure medications to take during pregnancy.

WHAT DOES IT ALL MEAN?

- ACE inhibitors are a class of oral medications commonly used to treat high blood pressure.

- These medications are particularly effective at slowing kidney disease in people with diabetes.
- Cough is a side effect of ACE inhibitors that may require switching to another class of blood pressure medications (that is, ARBs).
- People using ACE inhibitors should have their kidney function and potassium levels monitored regularly.

Angiotensin-Receptor Blockers

Angiotensin-receptor blockers (ARBs) are oral blood pressure medications. A ACE inhibitors are often the preferred treatment for people with diabetes who ha blood pressure and the early stages of diabetic kidney disease with albuminuria of these medications are also approved to treat heart failure in people with diab used after a heart attack.

▶ WHAT YOU NEED TO KNOW

What Are ARBs?

These medications are available as oral tablets. ARBs are manufactured under different brand names. These are the most common:

- Candesartan (brand name Atacand)
- Irbesartan (brand name Avapro)
- Losartan (brand name Cozaar)
- Olmesartan (brand name Benicar)
- Telmisartan (brand name Micardis)
- Valsartan (brand name Diovan)

What Do They Do?

Angiotensin II is a hormone that constricts blood vessels and leads to salt ar retention in the body. This results in higher blood pressure. ARBs prevent angiote from binding to its receptor; hence these effects do not occur. These medications similar effect to ACE inhibitors, which block the production of angiotensin II.

How Are They Taken?

Each ARB is taken in a different dosage and frequency. The treatment plan wi for each person; consult your health care provider for more information.

Facts about ARBs:

- ARBs are effective at controlling blood pressure.

- ARBs are especially useful for treating people with diabetes who have albuminuria and to prevent the progression of kidney disease.
- People who experience a cough when taking ACE inhibitors usually do not have this side effect when taking ARBs.
- People who take ARBs need to have regular blood tests to check their kidney function and potassium levels.

Warning!

- ARBs should not be taken with ACE inhibitors—the combination increases the risk of low blood pressure, high potassium levels, and kidney problems.
- Pregnant women should *not* take ARBs. These medications have been shown to harm the unborn baby. Talk to your health care provider about alternative medications to take during pregnancy.

WHAT DOES IT ALL MEAN?

- ARBs are common medications used to treat high blood pressure and to slow the progression of diabetic kidney disease in those with albuminuria.
- ARBs may be used instead of an ACE inhibitor in those that develop a cough, as ARBs do not usually have this side effect.
- People using ARBs should have their kidney function and potassium levels monitored regularly.

Beta-Blockers

Beta-blockers are medications used to treat a range of conditions, including hypertension (high blood pressure). Beta-blockers are recommended for people with diabetes who have high blood pressure, especially those who have a history of heart attack. These medications are also used to treat many other conditions, including heart failure, chest pain from heart disease (*angina*), and certain irregular heart rhythms (*arrhythmias*).

▶ WHAT YOU NEED TO KNOW

What Are Beta-Blockers?

These medications are available as oral tablets. Beta-blockers are often prescribed in generic form. These are some of the most common:

- Atenolol (brand name Tenormin)

- Carvedilol (brand name Coreg)
- Labetalol (common brand names include Trandate, Normodyne)
- Metoprolol (common brand names include Lopressor, Toprol)
- Propranolol (common brand names include Inderal, Hemangeol, Innopran)

What Do They Do?

Beta-blockers bind to a molecule known as the *beta-receptor* on nerves in the heart, blocking the hormones norepinephrine and epinephrine (adrenaline) from binding to the receptor. Thus, the heart beats less forcibly and more slowly, which lowers the blood pressure. Slowing the heartbeat also reduces the risk of arrhythmias and can improve heart function in those with heart failure.

How Are They Taken?

Each beta-blocker is taken in a different dosage and frequency. The treatment plan will differ for each person; consult your health care provider for more information.

Facts about Beta-Blockers

- People taking beta-blockers might not feel the warning signs of low blood glucose, such as trembling or heart palpitations. This can sometimes lead to unrecognized drops in blood glucose levels without warning.
- There is a slight risk that beta-blockers could increase blood glucose levels, but the long-term benefits of controlling your blood pressure far outweigh this low risk.
- People with kidney or liver problems should consult their providers before taking beta-blockers.
- Beta-blockers are often a preferred medication to lower blood pressure in those with a history of heart disease or heart failure.

Warning!

- People who take insulin or sulfonylureas should always consult their health care provider or pharmacist before taking beta-blockers because these drugs may mask symptoms of low blood glucose levels.
- Talk to your health care provider if you are pregnant before taking these medications.

WHAT DOES IT ALL MEAN?

- Beta-blockers are effective medications to reduce blood pressure, especially in those with a history of heart disease.

- Beta-blockers may hide certain symptoms of hypoglycemia, such as sweating and shakiness, so caution must be used.

Calcium Channel Blockers

Calcium channel blockers are medications that treat hypertension and arrhythmias. Certain calcium channel blockers might also slow down kidney damage from diabetes.

▶ WHAT YOU NEED TO KNOW

What Are Calcium Channel Blockers?

Calcium channel blockers are available as oral tablets and manufactured under several different brand names. These are the most common:

- Amlodipine (brand name Norvasc)
- Nifedipine (common brand names Procardia, Adalat)

Diltiazem (common brand names Cardizem, Dilt-CD, Tiazac) and verapamil (common brand names Verelan, Calan, Covera-HS) are calcium channel blockers that are not routinely used to treat high blood pressure but may slow kidney damage in people with early stages of diabetic kidney disease.

What Do Calcium Channel Blockers Do?

Calcium normally flows through channels in and out of the cells in the body. Calcium channel blockers block these so that calcium enters the cells more slowly in blood vessels or the heart. With less calcium, the blood vessels and the heart relax, and the blood pressure is lowered.

How Are They Taken?

Each type of calcium channel blocker is taken in a different dosage and frequency. The treatment plan will differ for each person; consult your health care provider for more information.

Facts about Calcium Channel Blockers

- There are two classes of calcium channel blockers: one that primarily reduces heart rate (verapamil and diltiazem) and others that primarily reduce blood pressure (amlodipine and nifedipine).
- Certain calcium channel blockers can also slow the progression of kidney disease in people with protein in their urine. If people cannot tolerate ACE inhibitors or ARBs, they may be prescribed a calcium channel blocker (such as verapamil or diltiazem) for diabetic kidney disease.

- Calcium channel blockers are generally safe to use in people with kidney problems.
- People with liver problems should consult their health care provider before taking calcium channel blockers, as some may be used with caution in lower doses.
- Constipation and fluid retention are common side effects of calcium channel blockers.

Warning!
- Talk to your health care provider if you are pregnant before taking these medications.

- Calcium channel blockers are effective blood pressure-lowering medications for people with diabetes.
- Some calcium channel blockers can also slow the progression of diabetic kidney disease.

Diuretics

Diuretics are medications that remove fluid from the body. Diuretics are recommended for individuals with diabetes who have high blood pressure. Some diuretics are also used in people with heart failure or excess fluid in the body, called *edema*.

▶ WHAT YOU NEED TO KNOW

What Are Diuretics?

Most diuretics are taken by mouth, though injectable versions exist for some (typically for use in the hospital). Some common oral versions include the following:
- Hydrochlorothiazide (marketed as Microzide and others)
- Chlorothiazide (brand name Diuril)
- Spironolactone (brand name Aldactone)
- Furosemide (brand name Lasix)
- Chlorthalidone (brand name Thalitone)
- Amiloride (brand name Midamor)
- Triamterene (brand name Dyrenium)

What Do They Do?

Diuretics work in the kidney, an organ that normally produces urine and balances the amounts of salt and water in the body. Diuretics work by helping more sodium enter the urine, which takes water with it and removes extra salt and water from the body, decreasing blood pressure.

How Are They Taken?

Each type of diuretic is taken in a different dosage and frequency. The treatment plan will differ for each person; consult your health care provider for more information.

Facts about Diuretics

- Diuretics are often added to combination pills that contain ACE inhibitors, ARBs, or other blood pressure medications. That way, people can take multiple medications in a single pill.
- Diuretics are generally safe to use in people with liver problems. Because diuretics work in the kidneys, these drugs may become less effective in people with advanced kidney disease.
- Diuretics can occasionally lead to imbalances in the amount of salt or potassium in the body. People should have regular blood tests to monitor their kidney function and potassium and sodium levels.

Warning!

- Talk to your health care provider if you are pregnant before taking these medications.

WHAT DOES IT ALL MEAN?

- Diuretics are medications that remove salt and water from the body.
- Diuretics are used to treat hypertension in people with diabetes.
- Electrolytes (such as sodium and potassium) must be monitored when taking diuretics.

MEDICATIONS FOR CHOLESTEROL ABNORMALITIES
Statins

Statins are medications used to treat cholesterol abnormalities (*dyslipidemia*). They are widely used in people with diabetes and have been shown to reduce the risk of heart attack and stroke and to prevent early death. These medications work by mainly lowering LDL (bad) cholesterol as well as triglycerides and raising HDL (good) cholesterol.

▶ WHAT YOU NEED TO KNOW

What Are Statins?

These medications are available as oral tablets. Several types of statins are available, including the following:

- Atorvastatin (brand name Lipitor)
- Fluvastatin (brand name Lescol)
- Lovastatin (brand name Altocor)
- Pravastatin (brand name Pravachol)
- Rosuvastatin (brand name Crestor)
- Simvastatin (brand name Zocor)

How Do They Work?

Statins prevent the formation of cholesterol by blocking an enzyme (HMG CoA reductase) in the liver that normally helps build more cholesterol.

How Are They Taken?

Your health care provider will create a treatment regimen to best serve your needs. In general:

- **Atorvastatin** Between 10 to 80 milligrams (mg), taken once daily
- **Fluvastatin** Between 20 to 80 mg, taken once daily, usually at bedtime, or Fluvastatin XL 80 mg, taken once daily
- **Lovastatin** Between 20 to 80 mg, taken once daily, usually at bedtime
- **Pravastatin** Between 10 to 80 mg, taken once daily
- **Rosuvastatin** Between 5 to 40 mg, taken once daily
- **Simvastatin** Between 10 to 40 mg, taken once daily, usually at bedtime

Facts about Statins

- Statins are effective LDL cholesterol–lowering medications. In most people these drugs lower total and LDL cholesterol by 10% to 50%, lower triglycerides by about 20% to 40%, and raise good HDL cholesterol by about 5% to 10% depending on the specific medication and dose.
- The benefits of statins extend beyond their effect of lowering cholesterol. They have other effects that can prevent heart attacks and stroke in people with diabetes, possibly due to reducing inflammation in the body.
- Your provider will likely monitor liver function periodically while taking these medications. Some studies have suggested that statins may increase

the risk of getting diabetes or worsen existing diabetes. However, these risks are small, and the benefits of statins far outweigh this possible adverse effect.

- In very rare cases, statins can cause severe muscle aches. If this side effect occurs, contact your health care provider. This is more likely to occur in people who take statins together with other cholesterol medications called *fibric acid derivatives*, specifically gemfibrozil.

Warning!

- Statins are harmful to the fetus and are not to be used during pregnancy under any circumstances.

WHAT DOES IT ALL MEAN?

- Statins are highly effective at lowering LDL cholesterol.
- These drugs also lower the risk of heart attack and stroke in people with diabetes, even in those without high cholesterol levels, due to their wide-ranging effects in the body.
- Most people with diabetes, especially those with other risk factors for heart disease, benefit from statin use.
- It may take several weeks or months to see the full effects of statin therapy on cholesterol levels.

Ezetimibe

Ezetimibe is a drug used to treat high LDL cholesterol, including in people with inherited diseases of high cholesterol.

▶ WHAT YOU NEED TO KNOW

What Is Ezetimibe?

This medication is available as an oral tablet (brand name Zetia).

What Does It Do?

This drug prevents the digestive tract from absorbing cholesterol into the body.

How Is It Taken?

- Ezetimibe is usually taken by mouth once daily.
- Most people take 10 mg per day, but your exact dose will be determined by your health care provider.

- Often, ezetimibe is taken with statins.

Facts about Ezetimibe
- Ezetimibe lowers LDL cholesterol by 15% to 20%.
- This medication causes very few side effects when taken without other medications. In rare cases, people have reported dizziness and joint pain.

Warning!
- Talk to your health care provider if you are pregnant before using this medication.

WHAT DOES IT ALL MEAN?
- Ezetimibe is an oral medication used to treat high LDL cholesterol.
- It is almost always used in combination with statin drugs. Sometimes it is used alone in people who don't tolerate statin drugs to lower LDL levels.

Niacin

Niacin is a medication typically used to increase levels of HDL, or "good cholesterol."

▶ WHAT YOU NEED TO KNOW

What Is Niacin?
Niacin is used to treat people with low levels of HDL (good cholesterol) and can increase levels by 15% to 35%. It can also lower levels of LDL (bad cholesterol) by 10% to 20% but to a lesser degree than other medications (such as statins). In some people it can lower triglycerides by up to 50%.

What Does It Do?
Niacin is a B vitamin that prevents the breakdown of HDL particles, therefore increasing their numbers. Niacin also prevents the release of fatty acids and reduces their levels in the blood. This prevents the formation of triglycerides and LDL.

How Is It Taken?
These medications are taken as oral tablets. The following are some common forms:
- Immediate-acting niacin (brand name Niacor; an over-the-counter version is marketed as Niacin)

- Extended-release niacin (brand name Niaspan ER)
- Over-the-counter slow-release niacin (brand name Slo-niacin)
- Sustained-release niacin (brand name Niacin SR)

Facts about Niacin
- Niacin is currently the most effective drug to boost levels of HDL.
- Despite an improvement in cholesterol, most studies of niacin have not shown lower rates of heart disease or stroke.
- Niacin can cause multiple side effects, some of which are serious, such as gastrointestinal or other bleeding, stomach ulcers, and liver damage.
- Some people taking niacin experience flushing (redness) and warmth in their face, neck, and arms, especially after eating hot drinks or food. People can prevent this side effect by taking an aspirin (check with your provider regarding dose) 30 minutes before taking niacin, if they are also prescribed aspirin. Niaspan ER, a slow-release form of the drug, causes this side effect less often than other forms of niacin.
- Niacin should be used with caution in people with kidney disease.
- Niacin should not be used in people with active liver disease.

Warning!
- Talk to your health care provider if you are pregnant before taking this medication.

WHAT DOES IT ALL MEAN?

- Niacin is a medication that can raise HDL cholesterol, lower LDL cholesterol, and lower triglycerides.
- The most common side effect, flushing, occurs in up to half of people. This can be reduced by taking aspirin prior to niacin and should improve over time.
- Because of possible side effects and a lack of clear evidence about whether it is beneficial for reducing heart attacks or stroke, niacin is not commonly prescribed as a first-line medication in people with abnormal cholesterol levels.

Omega-3 Fatty Acids

Omega-3 fatty acids are found in high concentrations in fish oil. They lower triglyceride levels in the blood.

What Are Omega-3 Fatty Acids?

Omega-3 fatty acids are a certain type of fat found in high concentrations in fish oil. They can be taken by either eating large amounts of cold-water fish or by taking supplements. They are also found in plant oils (such as flaxseed, soybean, or canola oils), walnuts, chia seeds, and other foods (for example, eggs) fortified in omega-3s.

What Do They Do?

Along with a healthy diet, omega-3 fatty acid medications can lower triglyceride levels by up to 50% in people with very high triglyceride levels. Omega-3 fatty acids are needed for normal body metabolism. Since the body does not produce its own omega-3 fatty acids, they can only be obtained from food or supplements. They may also reduce inflammation.

How Are They Taken?

Omega-3 fatty acids are found in cold-water fish (such as salmon and mackerel), but most people take them through oral supplements. Generic and prescription-strength fish oils are available (brand names Lovaza, Vascepa, Epanova, and Omtryg) that require taking 2 or 4 grams per day. However, there are many over-the-counter fish oil dietary supplements manufactured as well.

Facts about Omega-3 Fatty Acids

- Fish oils, containing omega-3 fatty acids, are sold in most supermarkets, drug stores, and health food stores. Most are available over the counter, but your provider may order prescription-strength fish oils that deliver a potent dose of omega-3.
- Most people take fish oils without experiencing side effects, but some have reported a fishy taste in the mouth, feeling slightly nauseated, or burping more than usual. If this happens, look for fish oil supplements that have a special coating to aid digestion—this is usually advertised on the label. Additionally, fish oil capsules can be frozen to reduce this side effect.
- Although they lower triglyceride levels, fish oils have not been proven to reduce the risk of heart attacks, stroke, heart failure, or death in people without a history of cardiovascular disease.
- Few scientific studies have explored how fish oil supplements interact with other drugs. For that reason, it's important to tell your health care provider which nutritional supplements you're taking.

- Fish oil may increase bleeding in people who are taking aspirin, clopidogrel (brand name Plavix), or blood thinners such as warfarin (see "Anticoagulants" on page 287). Speak to your provider before you take fish oil supplements, especially if you are taking any of these medications.

Warning!
- Talk to your health care provider if you are pregnant before taking this medication.

WHAT DOES IT ALL MEAN?
- Omega-3 fatty acids, found in fish oils, can lower blood triglyceride levels by up to 50%.
- Omega-3 enriched eggs are also available.
- Vegetarian omega-3 supplements may contain different types of fatty acids.
- They are available both over the counter and as a prescription.

Fibric Acid Derivatives

Fibric acid derivatives (or *fibrates*) are typically used to treat people with either high triglycerides, low HDL, or elevated LDL cholesterol.

▶ **WHAT YOU NEED TO KNOW**

What Are Fibric Acid Derivatives?

Fibric acid derivatives are oral medications. Several fibric acid derivatives are available:
- Fenofibrate (common brand names Tricor, Lofibra, Fenoglide, Antara)
- Fenofibrate extended release (brand name Trilipix)
- Gemfibrozil (brand name Lopid)

What Do They Do?

Fibric acid derivatives work by speeding up the removal of triglycerides from the bloodstream. These medications also block the liver's production of very-low-density lipoprotein (VLDL), a protein that carries triglycerides in the blood.

How Are They Taken?

Each type of fibrate is taken in a different dosage and frequency. The treatment plan will differ for each person; consult your health care provider for more information.

Facts about Fibric Acid Derivatives
- These medications are highly effective and have been shown to lower triglycerides by 25% to 50%, raise HDL cholesterol by about 10% to 15%, and decrease LDL by 10% to 20%.
- Despite these beneficial effects on lipid levels, they have not been proven to reduce the risk of heart disease or stroke.
- Fibric acid derivatives should not be used in people with severe kidney disease.
- In some cases, fibric acid derivatives can cause abnormal liver test results.
- Some common side effects include abdominal cramps and upset stomach.
- Some people may have muscle aches while taking these drugs, but usually when they are also taking statin medications. In rare cases, this can progress to severe muscle pain and muscle breakdown, which can lead to kidney problems. This type of side effect is less likely when people take fenofibrate rather than gemfibrozil.

Warning!
Talk to your health care provider if you are pregnant before taking this medication.

WHAT DOES IT ALL MEAN?
- Fibric acid derivatives are effective in lowering high triglycerides, which in turn can lead to pancreatitis if left untreated (see "Pancreatitis" on page 149).
- Side effects are generally mild, but people taking statin medications should be aware of an increased risk of muscle pain with certain fibrates.

Bile Acid Sequestrants
Bile acid sequestrants are used to treat people with cholesterol abnormalities and can lower LDL. Colesevelam is a specific bile acid sequestrant used to lower blood glucose levels in people with type 2 diabetes.

▶ WHAT YOU NEED TO KNOW
What Are Bile Acid Sequestrants?
These medications are available as oral tablets or powders. The following are some common forms:
- Cholestyramine (brand name Questran) is an oral powder.

- Colestipol (brand name Colestid) comes in the form of granules or powder, which must be mixed with water or juice. This drug is also available in large tablets.
- Colesevelam (brand name Welchol) comes in an oral tablet.

What Do They Do?

The liver converts cholesterol to digestive fluids called *bile acids*. These drugs capture bile acids in the intestines and send them out of the body in the stool. The liver makes up for this loss by converting even more cholesterol to bile acids. Since more bile acid is lost in the stool, cholesterol in the body decreases. Scientists are still not sure how colesevelam lowers blood glucose.

How Are They Taken?

Each type of bile acid sequestrant is taken differently. The treatment plan will differ for each person; consult your health care provider for more information.

Facts about Bile Acid Sequestrants

- Bile acid sequestrants can lower LDL cholesterol by 10% to 20% and can mildly boost HDL.
- These drugs sometimes increase triglyceride levels and may not be appropriate for people who already have high levels.
- In general, bile acid sequestrants have not been proven to prevent heart disease or stroke.
- Colesevelam is approved for the treatment of diabetes, though the mechanism for this action is still unclear.
- Side effects often include constipation and sometimes gas or bloating.
- Bile acid sequestrants can cause problems with your stomach absorbing certain medications and vitamins, so talk to your health care provider about when to take these medications.

Warning!

- Consult your provider if you are also taking other drugs. You may need to adjust when you take your doses so that the bile acid sequestrants finish their work in the intestines before you take other medications or vitamins.
- These drugs should not be taken by people with a diagnosis of bowel obstructions or gastroparesis (slowed stomach emptying).

WHAT DOES IT ALL MEAN?

- Bile acid sequestrants can lower LDL.

- Colesevelam can also treat type 2 diabetes and lower blood glucose levels by up to 0.5%, or 5.5 millimoles per mole (mmol/mol), but is not widely used for this purpose.
- These drugs can interfere with the absorption of certain medications, so appropriate timing of these medications is important.

PCSK9 Inhibitors

PCSK9 inhibitors are injectable medications to treat people with inherited diseases of high cholesterol, as well as people with known heart disease or stroke who have high LDL cholesterol levels that cannot be managed with statins alone.

▶ WHAT YOU NEED TO KNOW

What Are PCSK9 Inhibitors?

These are injectable medications and include the following:

- Evolocumab (brand name Repatha)
- Alirocumab (brand name Praluent)

How Do They Work?

These drugs help remove cholesterol from the body. They are antibodies that shut down an enzyme called PCSK9, which normally limits the amount of cholesterol that can be removed from the blood. Blocking this enzyme allows the liver to remove more LDL cholesterol and send it out of the body.

How Are They Taken?

These medications are injections that can be given every 2 weeks or monthly. Talk to your health care provider about specific dosing recommendations.

Facts about PCSK9 Inhibitors

- These drugs can lower LDL cholesterol by up to 60%.
- PCSK9 inhibitors are very effective at lowering LDL and have been shown to reduce the risk of cardiovascular events (such as heart attacks or stroke) in people with a history of cardiovascular disease.
- These medications are only for people on the highest tolerated doses of statin medications who still need extra LDL cholesterol lowering.
- Some people taking evolocumab may experience flu-like symptoms, respiratory tract infections, back pain, or bruising at the injection site.
- Some people taking alirocumab have reported pain, itching, or bruising at the injection site. Others experience liver issues, which can be detected with a blood test.

Warning!
- Talk to your health care provider if you are pregnant before taking this medication.

WHAT DOES IT ALL MEAN?

- PCSK9 inhibitors are injectable medications that are very effective at lowering LDL.
- These medications are expensive and may require insurance approval before starting therapy.
- They are generally only used in people with a history of heart disease or stroke who are already on the highest tolerated dose of statins and need additional cholesterol lowering.

MEDICATIONS TO PREVENT CARDIOVASCULAR DISEASE
Anticoagulants

Anticoagulants are medications that prevent the formation of blood clots. They are used to treat people with a history of heart disease, stroke, or previous blood clots and to prevent blood clots from developing in people with an irregular heart rhythm called *atrial fibrillation*. These medicines are sometimes referred to as "blood thinners."

▶ **WHAT YOU NEED TO KNOW**

What Are Anticoagulants?

Several types of anticoagulants are available. Some of the most common ones taken by mouth include the following:
- Warfarin (brand name Coumadin) and direct oral anticoagulants (DOACs) are used to treat and prevent blood clots in the peripheral blood vessels (called *deep venous thrombosis*) and in the lungs (called *pulmonary embolism*). These clots can subsequently break apart and become lodged in a major blood vessel, disrupting blood flow to the brain (to cause a stroke) or block blood flow to the heart (to cause a heart attack). These medications reduce the formation of blood clots in people with atrial fibrillation. Coumadin can also be used to prevent another heart attack in people with a previous history.
- DOACs include the medications dabigatran (brand name Pradaxa), rivaroxaban (brand name Xarelto), apixaban (brand name Eliquis), and edoxaban (brand name Savaysa).

How Do They Work?

Anticoagulants "thin" the blood to reduce the chances of clot formation, which can cut off critical blood supply to parts of the heart and brain and to blood vessels in other parts of the body, such as the arms or legs.

Warfarin blocks the formation of *coagulation factors* in the blood that are needed to form clots. DOACs prevents some of these blood-clotting factors from working properly.

How Are They Taken?

Your health care provider will work with you to tailor a treatment regimen to your specific needs, but in general:

- Warfarin is dosed differently for each person, depending on many factors, and requires frequent blood-test monitoring called INR, or *international normalized ratio*. The typical daily dose ranges from 2 to 10 mg. The dose is adjusted every few weeks based on the INR until stable.
- DOACs are taken once or twice daily; talk to your health care provider about specific dosing instructions.

Facts about Anticoagulants

- Anticoagulants are effective at preventing blood clot formation.
- Anticoagulants are commonly used in people with atrial fibrillation, a condition in which the heart beat is irregular. Without anticoagulant treatment, this heart rhythm can lead to clot formation, which can cause strokes.
- Because they are so effective at preventing blood from clotting, anticoagulants can make it difficult to control a person's bleeding, even from a small cut.
- Bleeding from ulcers in the stomach or gastrointestinal tract are more common in people who use anticoagulants and can be life-threatening.
- Many drugs interact with warfarin and DOACs. People on these medications should ask their health care provider or pharmacist before taking other medications because drug interactions could cause their blood to become too thick or too thin.
- People taking warfarin should talk to their health care provider about keeping a consistent dietary intake of vitamin K (often found in green leafy vegetables) since this vitamin influences the medication's effectiveness.
- Do not stop taking a DOAC without discussing it with your provider and taking another anticoagulant in its place.

Warning!
- Warfarin should not be used during pregnancy.
- Talk to your health care provider if you are pregnant before taking any anticoagulant medication.

WHAT DOES IT ALL MEAN?

Anticoagulants, pills that "thin" the blood, are used to treat blood clots and to prevent blood clots from forming in the legs or lungs. If untreated, blood clots can cause a heart attack or stroke in people with diabetes. They should be taken as directed to allow them to work properly. Regular blood testing for INR is important for persons taking warfarin, so the correct dose can be selected. This will prevent clotting problems from a dose that is too low and bleeding problems from a dose that is too high.

Antiplatelet Medications

The body uses platelets to form clots and prevent bleeding. Antiplatelet medications block the function of platelets, leading to less clotting. This can be desirable for lowering the risk of heart attacks or strokes in certain people, particularly people with diabetes.

▶ WHAT YOU NEED TO KNOW

What Are Antiplatelet Medications?

Several types of antiplatelet medications are available. Some of the most common ones taken by mouth include the following:
- Aspirin is used to reduce the risk of a first heart attack or stroke in people at high risk of developing these conditions and to prevent repeated heart attacks and stroke in people with diabetes.
- Clopidogrel (brand name Plavix) is used to treat heart disease, stroke, or peripheral vascular disease and to prevent repeated heart attacks and stroke.

How Do They Work?

Some heart attacks and strokes occur as a result of small clots forming in the blood vessels that supply the heart or brain. This leads to a blockage that can prevent the blood supply from reaching these important organs. Aspirin and clopidogrel prevent platelets from sticking together and creating a blood clot. This can help prevent heart attacks and strokes.

How Are They Taken?

Your health care provider will work with you to tailor a treatment regimen to your specific needs, but in general:

- Aspirin is usually taken once a day; daily doses range from 75 to 325 mg.
- Clopidogrel is taken once a day; the daily dose is usually 75 mg.

Facts about Antiplatelet Drugs

- Because antiplatelet medications impair clotting, these medications can make it more difficult to control a person's bleeding.
- Bleeding from ulcers in the stomach or gastrointestinal tract are more common in people who use these drugs.
- Antiplatelet medications are commonly used after heart procedures that open blocked arteries in the heart, such as a coronary angioplasty or stent placement, to prevent a clot from occurring.

Warning!

- Aspirin should not be used during pregnancy.
- Talk to your health care provider if you are pregnant before taking any antiplatelet medication.

WHAT DOES IT ALL MEAN?

Antiplatelet medications are pills that work to prevent clot formation. These medicines can be used to prevent heart attacks and strokes in people with diabetes at high risk for these conditions, especially among those with a previous history. People taking these medications may be at risk for having bleeding complications.

Chapter 11

DIABETES TECHNOLOGY AND EQUIPMENT

Glucose Meters

Glucose meters are handheld devices that enable you to test your blood glucose levels at home. Using a small lancing device to puncture the skin, usually from one of the fingers, you can get a tiny amount of blood. This small drop of blood is then put on a glucose test strip and placed in the glucose meter, which, within seconds, gives an accurate measure of the blood glucose level.

▶ **WHAT YOU NEED TO KNOW**

There are many things to consider when choosing a glucose meter (figure 11.1). Here are some steps that can help you decide which one is right for you.

Step One: Know Your Needs

If you are newly diagnosed with diabetes—or if you have trouble keeping your blood glucose levels in the target range and have frequent changes to your treatment regimen—a glucose meter with more advanced features may be right for you. If you are on multiple daily injections of insulin, you will likely need to check your blood glucose multiple times each day, such as before meals and at bedtime.

On the other hand, if your blood glucose level is well managed and you are not taking insulin or other medications that can cause low blood glucose levels, then you might need to check less frequently (for example, daily before breakfast) or only on occasion when you are not feeling well. You also might not require a model with as many advanced features. A simple, basic glucose meter may fit your needs.

Step Two: Know the Available Features

Most glucose meters give readings in 5 seconds or less, and most can store at least 3 months of results for download to a computer. Some meters send the glucose result directly to an insulin pump or connect with a smartphone. Most meters are small and portable and thus easy to take on the go. Other meters have large print numbers that are ideal for individuals with poor vision. There are even meters that report the glucose value aloud, so people who can't see as well can instead hear their glucose level after checking it.

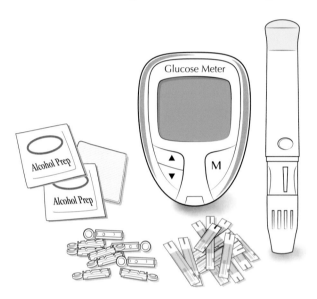

11.1 A glucose meter is a handheld device. Using a lancet and a lancing device to prick, a drop of blood is obtained from the fingertip. The blood is placed on a test strip inserted into the glucose meter. Most meters report a glucose value in a few seconds. © 2018, Johns Hopkins University, Art as Applied to Medicine

Step Three: Covering the Cost

Testing your blood glucose level can get expensive, especially if you need to test it several times a day. The cost of blood glucose meters is relatively low. However, the cost of test strips can be high and varies depending on the glucose meter you choose. Some strips cost up to $1 each, which can get expensive over time.

The good news is that if you have diabetes, your insurance will usually help cover the cost of your testing supplies, and there are many glucose meter options to choose from. For those with limited coverage, some discount stores sell meters and strips at a lower cost, but always check with your provider first to ensure their reliability.

Step Four: Reliable Results

Meters can only provide reliable results if they are used according to directions. It is crucial that your fingers are dry and free of foreign substances such as moisturizers, creams, or even food, all of which might cause falsely high or low readings. While fingertip testing is usually preferred, blood glucose levels can also be checked less commonly at other sites on the arms and legs. Even the least-expensive glucose meters are usually very accurate and reliable, but every meter needs to be tested for accuracy periodically. Your glucose meter will come with a set of bottles that contain specified amounts of glucose in so-called control solutions. Any time you start a new box of glucose test strips, or whenever your test results seem unusual, try taking a reading using the control solution. If the control solution does not give a result within the range that's listed on the bottle, it might be time to purchase a new meter or test strips. Other reasons for unreliable results include test strips that are expired or not stored properly. Never reuse or purchase used test strips.

WHAT DOES IT ALL MEAN?

Glucose meters are handheld devices that use a small drop of blood from your finger to measure blood glucose levels in seconds. Some meters can be used to test glucose in other less-common places, such as your arms or legs. These devices can be very valuable if you begin taking new medicines that can cause wide changes in blood glucose values, if you are on medications that can cause low blood glucose levels, or if you want to see if you are meeting your diabetes goals. There are a wide array of options available among different meters, but it is important to use them properly to get accurate results. Talk to your health care provider about what features may be most useful for you and how often and when you should test your blood glucose levels at home.

Continuous Glucose Monitors

Continuous glucose monitors (CGMs) are devices that use a sensor inserted under the skin to monitor interstitial glucose levels (glucose in the fluid surrounding the tissue that lies below your skin) frequently throughout the day. These levels reflect the blood glucose levels obtained through finger sticks or a laboratory blood draw, but there is a short time lag. A transmitting device sends informa-

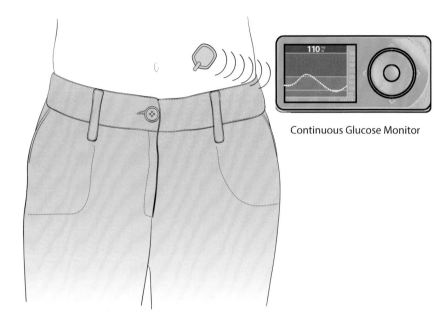

Continuous Glucose Monitor

11.2 A continuous glucose monitor uses a sensor inserted just below the skin to monitor glucose values. The values are transmitted to a handheld monitor, smartphone, or insulin pump and provide frequent information on glucose trends. © 2018, Johns Hopkins University, Art as Applied to Medicine

tion from the sensor to a receiver, which can be an external handheld monitor, smartphone, or insulin pump, that displays the glucose reading. The receiver also shows the direction and rate of change of the glucose, referred to as *the glucose trend*, and alerts you if the glucose level is going out of your preset target range.

▶ WHAT YOU NEED TO KNOW

CGMs provide additional information about blood glucose level trends compared to a finger stick, which only provides a snapshot. This is a device that can help people with diabetes manage their disease. The monitor can reveal the daily fluctuations in glucose levels in real time by providing an estimate of the glucose level every 5 to 15 minutes. In addition to letting you know where your glucose is now, it also lets you know where it is going and how fast it is changing (figure 11.2). If you have difficult-to-manage diabetes on insulin therapy—especially if you've had troublesome drops in blood glucose—your health care provider may suggest a CGM.

Who Should Wear CGMs?

The monitors may be especially helpful for

- persons with type 1 diabetes who have widely fluctuating glucose levels and have A1C levels higher than goal;
- persons with type 1 diabetes on insulin therapy who have good A1C levels but may be at risk for low blood glucose levels, particularly at night;
- persons with diabetes who experience frequent drops in blood glucose or low blood glucose levels so often that they no longer recognize the warning signs (called *hypoglycemia unawareness*); or
- persons with type 1 diabetes or insulin-treated type 2 diabetes who are motivated to use the feedback from a CGM to improve their diabetes management and get closer to goal.

How Do the Monitors Work?

A small sensor is placed beneath the skin, usually in the abdomen or the arm, using a needle insertion device. On top of the skin sits a transmitter that relays information to an external wireless handheld receiver, a smartphone, or an insulin pump.

Every 5 to 15 minutes, the sensor measures interstitial fluid glucose levels. The transmitter continuously sends the reading to a receiver or an insulin pump. The person with diabetes can see the results on the receiver's display screen, receive alerts, and download the information.

The two major CGM manufacturers in the United States as of 2018 are Dexcom and Medtronic. Newer "flash" CGMs, such as those manufactured by Abbott, provide glucose readings on demand when a scanner is placed over the sensor and do not require routine calibration with finger-stick readings from a glucose meter. CGMs can also offer the ability to monitor glucose readings directly on a smartphone. Remote real-time monitoring of glucose readings by family members and the ability to be alerted when the person is out of range are possible with many systems. A CGM developed by Senseonics that can last up to three months was also approved by the FDA in 2018. This CGM includes a pill-sized sensor implanted under the skin. A transmitter attached to the overlying skin then sends glucose readings to a smartphone.

How Well Do CGMs Work?

CGMs provide a huge amount of information—glucose measurements every few minutes all day, every day, for up to a week—but this information reflects the amount of glucose in the fluid just under the skin rather than the amount of glucose in the blood. The results are not as timely as home self-monitored blood glucose test meters. There is a small time lag (5 to 15 minutes), which means the reading from the CGM will run behind the true blood glucose level, which is important if the blood glucose level is changing rapidly. While blood glucose levels from finger sticks have been regarded as more accurate than from CGM, the accuracy of CGM systems is steadily improving, and the best systems now approximate the accuracy of some home blood glucose meters. Historically, the CGM could not serve as a replacement for regular home blood glucose testing in making treatment decisions, but some of the newer CGMs no longer require the results to be confirmed by finger-stick testing using a blood glucose meter before administering insulin. However, most CGMs will still need to be cross-checked for accuracy with results from a finger-stick glucose reading two or more times throughout the day.

WHAT DOES IT ALL MEAN?

- The vast amount of information gleaned from CGMs and the ability to immediately alert a person when his or her glucose levels are going out of target range can help modify a diabetes regimen.
- CGMs can be useful for people to explore how their blood glucose levels change during the day, particularly in response to eating and physical activity. They can also help monitor wide fluctuations in glucose in those with type 1 diabetes and are particularly useful to avoid low blood glucose levels at night.
- Some people wear CGMs for short periods of time (less than 72 hours) while others may wear them daily; the frequency of use depends on many factors and should be discussed with the health care provider.

Using an Insulin Pump to Manage Diabetes

Insulin pumps are small devices that deliver rapid-acting insulin through a catheter under the skin to people with type 1 diabetes (and sometimes type 2 diabetes) who would otherwise require multiple daily insulin injections. Pumps supply a low rate of preprogrammed insulin continuously to keep glucose levels steady while people are fasting and can deliver insulin boluses before meals and correct high glucose levels when instructed by the user (figure 11.3).

▶ WHAT YOU NEED TO KNOW

Insulin pumps have been around since the 1970s. Insulin pumps are most often used by those with type 1 diabetes and, in some cases, by those with insulin-treated type 2 diabetes. Depending on the brand and model, the insulin pump may hold up to 300 units of insulin or more. Some glucose meters share information with pumps wirelessly but still require input from the wearer before delivering insulin.

Insulin Pumps: Are You a Good Candidate?

Have you considered using an insulin pump? Some people with type 1 diabetes prefer pumps because they reduce the need for multiple daily injections of insulin.

Unfortunately, insulin pumps don't reduce the need for carbohydrate counting or glucose monitoring. People with type 1 diabetes still need to be aware of the insulin needed to cover their food intake and correct high blood glucose by pressing buttons on the pump to deliver the appropriate amount of insulin.

How Well Do Insulin Pumps Work?

Insulin pumps work best when people are motivated to use them correctly. While some pumps come equipped with blood glucose monitors that wirelessly send data to the pump, these monitors cannot actually determine the amount of insulin that the pump boluses to cover meals or high glucose levels. It is up to the user to decide how much insulin to give for meals based on the blood glucose level. Newer pumps integrated with CGMs are now available that analyze the glucose data provided by the CGM and automatically adjust the amount of background (basal) insulin delivered by the pump to both lower high glucose levels to target and prevent glucose levels from falling too low. However, users still need to input bolus insulin doses before meals. These newer pumps are called *closed hybrid-loop systems* (see "The Artificial Pancreas" on page 308).

People who use insulin pumps should check their blood glucose at least four times every day; the more regularly they check, the better the pump settings can be adjusted to effectively control blood glucose levels.

How Will I Know Which Model of Pump to Choose?

There are many types of insulin pumps on the market, all with different features (see "Types of Insulin Pump Devices" on page 299). This can seem overwhelming at first. Often the health care team (including the doctor, nurse, or diabetes educator) can recommend a specific model that will fit your personal needs.

How Are the Pumps Programmed?

When you first obtain an insulin pump, your health care provider will likely program settings into it based on your current insulin needs. The pump will

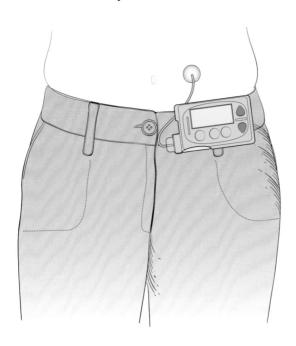

11.3 Insulin pumps are small devices that deliver insulin through a catheter just below the skin. The pumps deliver a continuous flow of "background," or basal insulin, to stabilize glucose values during fasting. In addition, using the amount of carbohydrates in a meal and the blood glucose value, a bolus of insulin can be calculated and given at mealtimes. © 2018, Johns Hopkins University, Art as Applied to Medicine

deliver a constant, steady infusion of insulin throughout the day to keep your blood glucose levels in a target range when you're not eating. This is the *basal rate*. When you eat, you can use the pump to deliver a larger dose, or bolus, of insulin to cover the carbohydrates from your meal and to correct for high blood glucose levels before the meal. This requires pressing buttons before the meal.

Many pumps have a built-in calculator that makes it easier for people to determine how much insulin they need to give themselves before a meal. These pumps can be programmed with the person's insulin-to-carbohydrate ratio and insulin sensitivity factor, so the user only needs to enter the number of carbohydrates in each meal and their current blood glucose level. The pump will do the math and guide the person on how much insulin to take.

Will I Wear the Pump All the Time?

In general, yes. However, some people remove the pump when they shower or plan to exercise for less than 60 minutes. Always check with your health care provider first. If you prefer to leave the pump on, you may need to eat a snack before or after exercising or adjust the pump's settings to reduce the infusion rate of insulin. Remember to revert to the pump's normal settings after your workout; some people may need lower settings for a few hours after exercise, as well.

What If the Pump Stops Working?

Before you start using a pump, it is very important to work with your health care team to learn what to do if the catheter comes out of your skin, if the pump stops working, or if an emergency arises.

Always have extra batteries and extra pump supplies on hand for the pump. Also make sure you have a reserve supply of syringes and long-acting injectable insulin in case you need to temporarily switch back to daily injections due to a pump malfunction.

If the pump stops delivering insulin for any reason, contact your pump's manufacturer and your health care provider for further instructions. You may need to temporarily take insulin injections until the pump is fixed. Follow the plan that your provider has prescribed for you.

WHAT DOES IT ALL MEAN?

Insulin pumps can be extremely useful when people are motivated to use them correctly. However, pumps do not take the place of counting carbs, checking blood glucose levels regularly, and calculating the proper dose of insulin before meals. If you decide to use an insulin pump, make sure you work with a knowledgeable and experienced health care provider to determine the appropriate settings. Stay in close contact with your providers and make sure you know what to do in an emergency if the pump stops working.

Types of Insulin Pump Devices

Insulin pumps may help achieve better blood glucose control with less risk of hypoglycemia and can also be more convenient and flexible for some people with diabetes who require insulin treatment (figure 11.4). An important advantage of newer pumps is that they include programmable bolus calculators to assist in choosing the right dose of insulin for a meal, for a snack, or for the correction of high blood glucose. They can be programmed based on your individual needs by your health care provider.

▶ WHAT YOU NEED TO KNOW

Some of the common insulin pumps are described in the tables following; there are also others. The top table lists their basic characteristics, while the bottom table goes into more detail about the special features you'll find on each pump.

Table 11.1. Basic characteristics of common insulin pumps

PUMP NAME (COMPANY)	SIZE (INCHES)	WEIGHT (OUNCES)	DISPLAY	INSULIN DELIVERY METHOD	INSULIN RESERVOIR
Animas OneTouch Ping* *(Animas Corp.)*	3.3 × 2.0 × 0.9	3.7 (with battery and empty reservoir)	Color	Tube	200 units
Animas Vibe* *(Animas Corp.)*	3.3 × 2.0 × 0.9	3.7 (without battery and with empty reservoir)	Color	Tube	200 units
Dana Diabecare IIS *(Sooil Development)*	3.0 × 1.8 × 0.7	2.15 (with battery and full reservoir)	Monochrome	Tube	300 units
MiniMed Paradigm Revel *(Medtronic)*	2 × 3.7 × 0.8	3.5 (with battery and full reservoir)	Monochrome	Tube	300 units
MiniMed 530G system *(Medtronic)*	2 × 3.7 × 0.8	3.7 (with battery and full reservoir)	Monochrome	Tube	300 units

Pump (Manufacturer)	Dimensions (in)	Weight (oz)	Display	Tubing	Reservoir capacity
MiniMed 630G system (*Medtronic*)	2.1 × 3.8 × 1.0	(without battery and with empty reservoir)	Color	Tube	300 units
MiniMed 670G system (*Medtronic*)	2.1 × 3.8 × 1.0	3.7 (without battery and with empty reservoir)	Color	Tube	300 units
OmniPod (Insulet Corp.)	Pod: 1.5 × 2.1 × 0.6 Personal diabetes manager (PDM): 2.4 × 4.4 × 1.0	0.88 (with empty reservoir) 4.4 (with batteries)	PDM: Color	Tubeless	200 units
t:flex Pump (Tandem Diabetes Care)	3.1 × 2.0 × 0.8	4.05 (with battery and full reservoir)	Color touch screen	Tube	480 units
t:slim G4 Pump** (Tandem Diabetes Care)	3.1 × 2.0 × 0.6	3.95 (with battery and full reservoir)	Color touch screen	Tube	300 units
t:slim X2 Pump (Tandem Diabetes Care)	3.1 × 2.0 × 0.6	3.95 (with battery and full reservoir)	Color touch screen	Tube	300 units

*Animas exited the insulin pump market at the end of 2017. New insulin pumps from Animas are no longer available, but people currently using Animas pumps will receive technical and supply support from Medtronic.

**The t:slim X2 Pump replaces the t:slim G4 Pump, but the company will continue to service this pump for the duration of the warranty.

Table 11.2. Advanced features of common insulin pumps

PUMP NAME (COMPANY)	INTERACTS WITH GLUCOSE METER	INTERACTS WITH CONTINUOUS GLUCOSE MONITOR (CGM)	FOOD DATABASE	UNIQUE FEATURES
*Animas One Touch Ping** (Animas Corp.)	Yes. OneTouch Ping Meter/Remote	No	Yes. Stores up to 500 foods, with nutrition information software, allowing users to customize food database	Meter/remote allows wireless delivery of insulin within 10 feet of pump
*Animas Vibe** (Animas Corp.)	No	Yes. Dexcom G4	Yes. Stores up to 500 foods, with nutrition information software, allowing users to customize food database	Integrates with CGM
Dana Diabecare IIS (Sooil Development)	No	No	No	Icon-based interface Can use multiple languages
MiniMed Paradigm Revel (Medtronic)	Yes. Compatible with Bayer Contour Next Link	Yes. Enlite sensor communicates directly to pump	No	A stand-alone pump with capability to have combined CGM
MiniMed 530G system (Medtronic)	Yes. Compatible with Bayer Contour Next Link	Yes. Enlite sensor communicates directly to pump	No	Pump can suspend for up to 2 hours if the sensor glucose values go below a preset low level
MiniMed 630G system	Yes. Compatible with Bayer	Yes. Enlite sensor communicates directly to	No	Pump can suspend insulin for up to 2 hours if sensor glucose values

MiniMed 670G system (Medtronic)	Yes. Compatible with Bayer Contour Next Link	Yes. Guardian Sensor 3 communicates directly to pump	No	adjusts basal insulin delivery based on CGM glucose levels to maximize time in target range. Pump can suspend insulin for up to 2 hours if sensor glucose values go below a preset low level
OmniPod (Insulet Corp.)	Yes. Freestyle glucometer built into PDM	Yes	Yes. PDM has information on more than 1,000 common foods	Tubing-free design, remote PDM controls pod's insulin delivery and can be up to 5 feet away. Built-in glucose meter. Automated insertion
t:Flex (Tandem Diabetes Care)	No	No	No	Touch screen. Insulin reservoir is 480 units, helpful for people requiring large amounts of insulin
t:slim G4** (Tandem Diabetes Care)	No	Yes. Dexcom G4	No	Touch screen insulin pump that integrates with Dexcom G4 continuous glucose monitor
t:slim X2 (Tandem Diabetes Care)	No	Yes. Dexcom G5 or G6	No	Designed for software updates that will allow future additional features without requiring purchase of a new device

* Animas exited the insulin pump market at the end of 2017. New insulin pumps from Animas are no longer available, but people currently using Animas pumps will receive technical and supply support from Medtronic will be available until Fall 2019.

** The t:slim X2 Pump replaces the t:slim G4 Pump, but the company will continue to service this pump for the duration of the warranty.

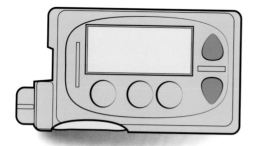

11.4 Several types of insulin pumps are available, each with different features.
© 2018, Johns Hopkins University, Art as Applied to Medicine

Insulin pumps are rapidly changing, and it is best to consult the individual company websites to check on the latest pump features (tables 11.1 and 11.2).

WHAT DOES IT ALL MEAN?

The tables provided can help you find a pump that best suits your lifestyle based on multiple characteristics. If you're unsure where to begin, take this list to your next appointment and ask your health care provider for help in narrowing down the best option for you.

Chapter 12

CUTTING-EDGE AND FUTURE TREATMENTS FOR DIABETES

Pancreas and Islet Transplantation

Pancreas or islet transplantations are surgical procedures that involve removing a whole pancreas (or only the part that makes insulin, called *islets*) from a deceased person and placing this tissue into a living person with type 1 diabetes (*allotransplant*) to correct high blood glucose levels and possibly eliminate the diabetes. Alternatively, when someone must have the pancreas removed for other medical conditions (such as pancreatitis), the islets from that pancreas may be separated and placed back into that same person (*autotransplant*) to keep blood glucose levels normal after the surgery.

▶ WHAT YOU NEED TO KNOW

Can Pancreas Transplants Cure Diabetes?

In this modern age of high-tech devices and groundbreaking therapies, people wonder if there are other ways of curing type 1 diabetes. After all, if your pancreas doesn't work, why not get a new one?

It is important to understand that the pancreas has two main functions. Its largest part, the exocrine pancreas, makes enzymes to break down food so it can be absorbed by the intestine. The much smaller portion, the endocrine pancreas, makes insulin and other hormones to help the body process food and use it for energy. Only the endocrine pancreas is deficient in autoimmune type 1 diabetes, so people with this disease need just the islets replaced, not the entire pancreas. However, it is difficult to separate the insulin-producing cells from the rest of the pancreas without damaging them.

As it turns out, organ transplants are recommended treatment options for

Table 12.1. Types of pancreas and islet transplantation

WHAT IS IT CALLED?	WHO IS IT FOR?	HOW IT WORKS	DRUGS T PREVENT O REJECTIC
Pancreas transplant alone (PTA)	People with frequent and severe drops in blood glucose	People receive a pancreas donated by a deceased person	Yes
Simultaneous pancreas and kidney transplant (SPK) or pancreas-after-kidney transplant	People with diabetes and severe kidney disease	The kidney and pancreas are transplanted together in SPK (most common). Sometimes the kidney transplant occurs first, then the pancreas transplant at a later date People receive a pancreas donated by a deceased person and a kidney donated by either a living or deceased donor	Yes
Islet allotransplantation	Only available to people with type 1 diabetes enrolled in certain research studies	Surgeons remove the insulin-releasing cells (islets) from a donor's pancreas and inject those islets into another person (via the portal vein of the liver)	Yes
Islet auto-transplantation	People with chronic pancreatitis who are having their entire pancreas removed for treatment of pain	Surgeons extract islets from the surgically removed pancreas and reinject those cells into the same person via the portal vein of the liver	No

certain people with type 1 diabetes. A few different types of transplants are available, depending on the need (table 12.1). The surgeon might replace the entire pancreas or just the islets responsible for releasing insulin from the pancreas. People who develop end-stage kidney disease as a complication of type 1 diabetes might opt for two new organs, transplanting both the kidney and the pancreas.

Organ Transplant Pros and Cons

An organ transplant can improve a person's enjoyment of life in many ways, but transplants are surgeries—and surgeries carry risks. It is important to carefully weigh the benefits of organ transplantation with all the possible risks before coming to a final decision. There are very few donors of pancreatic tissue because whereas a person can donate one of her or his two kidneys and still have normal kidney function, a living person generally cannot donate pancreatic tissue except in research studies. However, for those who do receive a deceased pancreas transplant alone, outcomes are steadily improving, and more than half these people may have good pancreatic function 5 years after the surgery.

A pancreas transplant can

- prevent wide and rapid fluctuations in blood glucose levels,
- eliminate diabetes or greatly simplify diabetes management, and
- reduce or eliminate the need for daily insulin injections.

But there are also serious risks:

- Risks of the surgery itself include infection; rarely, a heart attack or stroke during the procedure; and technical complications that prevent the surgery from going as smoothly as planned.
- The body will attack transplanted organs from another person because the immune system considers these foreign tissues to be a threat. The immune system in a person with type 1 diabetes will also attack the transplanted islet cells of the pancreas, just as it attacked the person's own islets years before. To reduce the chances of rejection after surgery, people who receive organ transplants must take immune-suppressing drugs for the rest of their lives. Unfortunately, these drugs also make people more susceptible to viral and bacterial infections and may increase blood glucose levels. They can also have other possible side effects, such as nerve or kidney damage.
- An islet allotransplant can correct high blood glucose levels and may eliminate diabetes in people with type 1 or reduce the amount of insulin they take every day. Similar to organ transplants, immune-suppressing drugs are needed for life. A total pancreatectomy with an islet autotransplant

in people with pancreatitis (see "Pancreatitis" on page 149) can prevent postsurgical diabetes, and immune-suppressing drugs are not needed. However, most people will require insulin injections again by 5 years after either type of islet transplant.

- Pancreas and islet transplants are only performed at specialized medical centers. Many people must travel far distances to find an experienced surgeon.

Great excitement surrounds the prospect of being able to grow insulin-producing cells in a laboratory, which would remove the need for donors. The cells could be implanted inside a special membrane to protect them from the immune system and therefore reduce the need for immune-suppressive medications. Studies of this technique are underway.

WHAT DOES IT ALL MEAN?

If you have extremely difficult to control type 1 diabetes, with or without kidney disease, or do not have diabetes but need to have your pancreas removed for other reasons, ask your health care provider about the possibility of a pancreas or islet transplant to prevent or reverse the symptoms of diabetes. For select people these transplants greatly reduce the need for daily insulin injections and lead to a more enjoyable life. Islet allotransplant for the cure of type 1 diabetes is still an experimental procedure limited to research settings.

The Artificial Pancreas

These days you can track almost anything with technology. Scientists are working on ways to make a small computer, such as your smartphone, act like a pancreas!

This "artificial pancreas" is actually an automated insulin-delivery system that uses several electronic devices. One device is a sensor that is inserted into the skin to track your blood glucose levels. The sensor sends information about blood glucose levels to your phone or other device, which has a sophisticated computer algorithm that triggers the insulin pump to deliver insulin as needed through a small tube in the skin. There are also efforts to develop a system that can give glucagon, a hormone that helps raise the blood glucose level when it is too low, in addition to the insulin.

Many of these automated systems are still being tested and are not yet available for purchase. But some currently available systems can prevent drops in blood glucose, especially during the night (see "Overnight Hypoglycemia" on page 43), while improving overall glucose management.

▶ WHAT YOU NEED TO KNOW

The Evolution of the Artificial Pancreas

The pump The first insulin pump was developed in the 1970s. Early insulin pumps were quite large and gradually became smaller until the 1980s and 1990s, when they could fit into the palm. These small pumps deliver short- or rapid-acting insulin at programmed rates throughout the day and can be commanded to deliver more insulin before meals or for spikes of blood glucose. However, they always require the user to control the amount of insulin released by pressing a button on the pump. These devices have been called *open-loop* pumps because no automatic feedback is sent to them.

The continuous glucose monitor Like the pump, the continuous glucose monitor (CGM) was developed in the 1970s and improved in the 1990s. However, this large system was meant for short-term use only, with results not visible to the person. New and improved versions monitor glucose levels continuously and report on them every 5 to 15 minutes using a sensor placed under the skin. They also alert the user to very high or low readings and to rapid changes in blood glucose levels. Examining trends in glucose levels can help guide the user in adjusting the insulin pump settings that control the delivery of insulin.

The computer In the theoretical artificial pancreas, an algorithm contained within a computer chip inside the pump analyzes glucose readings received from the CGM. The computer chip then automatically sends commands to the insulin pump to adjust the flow of insulin when glucose levels are falling too low or rising too high. This is a *closed-loop* system—that is, one that uses blood glucose data to continuously update the insulin delivery rates of the pump. Studies of early and partial artificial pancreas prototypes showed that low blood glucose levels (hypoglycemia) during sleep were reduced. In the United States, both the MiniMed 530 and 630G models have a combined insulin pump and CGM integrated in one device and offer an automated insulin shutoff feature (called *threshold-suspend*) when blood glucose levels run too low. The MiniMed 670G automatically lowers or increases the background insulin released by the pump throughout the day (that is, the basal rate) when the monitor predicts or detects glucose levels that are running too low or too high. Studies of the 670G have shown improvements in diabetes management leading to both a lowering of the A1C as well as less time spent with low blood glucose levels. However, this is called a *hybrid closed-loop* system since the pump is not fully automated, and the user must still press a button to administer insulin before meals.

So, What Is the Hold Up?

Hybrid closed-loop insulin pumps are now available to help correct blood glucose levels that are running too high or too low throughout the day. Many more brands of insulin pumps are being developed that will communicate with a CGM to help automate insulin delivery. Current systems do not yet automatically provide insulin for meals or adjust for exercise. This still requires the wearer to issue a meal bolus command or manually reduce insulin rates while exercising. In the future, more rapid-acting insulins and systems that can deliver glucagon along with insulin may help artificial pancreas systems to tightly regulate glucose levels and eventually take over more diabetes management from the user, including delivering insulin at mealtimes. The fully closed-loop insulin pump or artificial pancreas has yet to become a reality, but we are getting closer.

WHAT DOES IT ALL MEAN?

- The artificial pancreas is a yet-to-be-perfected device containing an insulin pump, a CGM, and a computer chip with an algorithm that reads glucose levels and instructs the insulin pump to automatically deliver insulin to keep blood glucose in a target range.
- Insulin pumps that have automatically adjusted basal rates or an automatic shutoff feature based on blood glucose readings are currently available and have been shown to improve diabetes management while reducing the amount of time a person spends with low glucose levels.
- Such technology should continue to improve into the future and could help people with type 1 diabetes (and some people with type 2 or other forms of diabetes) better manage their disease and perhaps improve their quality of life.

Appendix

DIABETES MEDICATIONS CURRENTLY AVAILABLE IN THE UNITED STATES

DRUG CLASS	GENERIC NAMES	BRAND NAMES
Short- or rapid-acting insulins	Aspart	Novolog, Fiasp
	Lispro	Humalog, Admelog
	Glulisine	Apidra
	Regular human insulin	Novolin R Humulin R
	Inhaled insulin	Afrezza
Intermediate- or long-acting insulins	Glargine	Lantus Basaglar Toujeo
	Detemir	Levemir
	NPH	Humulin N Novolin N
	Degludec	Tresiba

DRUG CLASS	GENERIC NAMES	BRAND NAMES
Premixed insulins	70% human insulin isophane suspension and 30% human insulin injection (NPH–regular 70/30 premix)	Novolin 70/30 Humulin 70/30
	70% insulin aspart protamine suspension and 30% insulin aspart injection (insulin aspart 70/30 premix)	Novolog Mix 70/30
	75% insulin lispro protamine suspension and 25% insulin lispro injection (insulin lispro 75/25 premix)	Humalog Mix 75/25
	50% insulin lispro protamine suspension and 50% insulin lispro injection (insulin lispro 50/50 premix)	Humalog Mix 50/50
Biguanides	Metformin	Glucophage
	Metformin XR (extended release)	Glucophage XR Fortamet Glumetza
Sulfonylureas	Glimepiride	Amaryl
	Glipizide	Glucotrol Glucotrol XL
	Glyburide	DiaBeta Micronase Glynase
Glinides	Repaglinide	Prandin
	Nateglinide	Starlix

Thiazolidinediones	Pioglitizone	Actos
	Rosiglitazone	Avandia
DPP-4 inhibitors	Sitaglitpin	Januvia
	Saxagliptin	Onglyza
	Linagliptin	Tradjenta
	Alogliptin	Nesina
Alpha-glucosidase inhibitors	Acarbose	Precose
	Miglitol	Glyset
Bile acid sequestrants	Colesevelam	Welchol
Dopamine agonists	Bromocriptine	Cycloset
Amylin mimetics	Pramlintide acetate	Symlin
GLP-1 agonists	Exenatide	Byetta
	Exenatide ER (extended release)	Bydureon
	Liraglutide	Victoza
	Semaglutide	Ozempic
	Dulaglutide	Trulicity
	Lixisenatide	Adlyxin
SGLT2 inhibitors	Canagliflozin	Invokana
	Dapagliflozin	Farxiga
	Empagliflozin	Jardiance

DRUG CLASS	GENERIC NAMES	BRAND NAMES
Oral combination pills	Pioglitazone & metformin	Actoplus Met
	Pioglitazone & glimepiride	Duetact
	Glyburide & metformin	Glucovance
	Glipizide & metformin	Metaglip
	Sitagliptin & metformin (XR)	Janumet Janumet XR
	Saxagliptin & metformin XR	Kombiglyze XR
	Linagliptin & metformin	Jentadueto
	Alogliptin & metformin	Kazano
	Alogliptin & pioglitazone	Oseni
	Repaglinide & metformin	Prandimet
	Rosiglitazone & metformin	Avandamet
	Rosiglitazone & glimepiride	Avandaryl
	Empagliflozin & linagliptin	Glyxambi
	Empagliflozin & metformin (XR)	Synjardy Synjardy XR
	Canagliflozin & metformin (XR)	Invokamet Invokamet XR
	Dapagliflozin & metformin XR	Xigduo XR
	Dapagliflozin & saxagliptin	Qtern
GLP-1 agonist/insulin combination injections	Insulin glargine & lixisenatide	Soliqua 100/33
	Insulin degludec & liraglutide	Xultophy 100/3.6

INDEX

artificial sweeteners, 90, *91*
aspartate aminotransferase enzyme, 148
aspirin therapy, 45, 108, 127, 289–90
atherosclerosis, 134
Atkins Diet, 92
atrial fibrillation, 287, 288
autoantibodies, 144, 193–96
autoimmune skin responses, 176
autonomic neuropathy, 166–68
autotransplant of islets, 305, *306*

bacterial infections, 178
balance training, 96
bariatric surgery, 102, 103–4
basal (intermediate- and long-acting)
    insulins: action of, *251, 252*; dosage and
    regimen for, 252–53; effectiveness and
    duration of effect of, *253*; overview of,
    250, *252, 311*
basal-bolus insulin injection therapy, 216
beta-blockers, 273–75
biguanides, 225, *312. See also* metformin
bile acid sequestrants, 284–85, *313*
bitter melon, 264
bladder disorders, 160–61, 167–68
blisters, 177
blood clots, 287–90
blood pressure, high. *See* hypertension
body mass index (BMI): calculating, 14,
    100–101; obesity and, 99; weight-loss
    surgery and, 103–4
bolus (short- and rapid-acting) insulins:
    converting to inhaled insulin units, *258*;
    effectiveness and duration of effect of,
    256; overview of, 254–57, *311*
bone mineral density test, 183
brain: dementia and neurodegenerative
    diseases, 108–10; depression, 80,
    110–12; function of, 2; strokes, 105–8
bromocriptine (Cycloset), 221, 245, *246,
    247, 313*

calcific shoulder periarthritis, 182–83
calcium channel blockers, 275–76

calories, 85
canagliflozin (Invokana), 221, 238, *313*
cancer, 187–90
candida, 196
carbohydrates, counting, 84, 85–87, 90
cardiologists, 129
cardiovascular disease: as cause of death,
    5; congestive heart failure, 127–29;
    diagnosis of, 127; dyslipidemia, 131–33,
    277–87; heart attacks, *126,* 126–27;
    hypertension, 129–31; medications to
    prevent, 287–90; metabolic syndrome,
    133–34; plaque in arteries, *125;* risk
    factors for, 124, 126; statins and, 278;
    symptoms of, 97
carpal tunnel syndrome, 181–82
cataracts, 115–16
celiac disease, 143–45
cellulitis, 197
Centers for Disease Control and Preven-
    tion (CDC), 19
cerebrovascular diseases, 105–8, *107*
certified diabetes educators, 82
cesarean deliveries, 206, 207–8
CGMs (continuous glucose monitors),
    293–96, *294,* 309
Charcot joint disease, 174–76
checkups, scheduling, 47
children with diabetes: MODY, 22–23;
    number of, 5; social support for, 51–52;
    type 2 diabetes in, 62–65
cholesterol, 131–32. *See also* dyslipidemia
cholinesterase inhibitors, 109
chromium, 264–65
cigarette smoking, *57,* 108, 127, 258
cinnamon, 265
cirrhosis, 146, 147
claudication, 135
closed hybrid-loop systems, 297, 309–10
closed-loop systems, 309
coagulation factors, 288
cocaine use, *57*
colesevelam (Welchol), 221, 250, 285,
    286, *313*

complementary and alternative treatments: herbs, supplements, and vitamins, 264–65; meditation and stress reduction, 266–68; overview of, 263–64

complex carbohydrates, 85

complications of diabetes: A1C level and risk of, 35; acute, 2; chronic, 2, 4; microvascular, 7, 9; overview of, 5; in persons with HIV, 69; small and large blood vessel, x. *See also specific organs*

congestive heart failure, 127–29, 244

continuous glucose monitors (CGMs), 293–96, *294*, 309

control solution for glucose meters, 293

coronary artery disease, 128

cortisol, 32

C-peptide test, *17*, 195

creatinine level, 155

critical leg ischemia, 135–36

cultural practices, 71, 73, 80

CYP3A4 inhibitors, 247

cystic fibrosis-related diabetes, 23–25

dapagliflozin (Farxiga), 221, 238, *313*

Da Qing study, 6

DASH (Dietary Approaches to Stop Hypertension) diet, 92

dawn phenomenon, 32–33

Dean Ornish Diet, 92

dementia, 108–10

dental care, 119–21

depression, 80, 110–12

Diabetes Control and Complications Trial, 7–8

Diabetes Prevention Program, 7, 19–20, 65

diabetes self-management education, 82–83

diabetic bullae, 177

diabetic dermopathy, 179

diabetic ketoacidosis (DKA), *17*, 35–37, 238–39

diabetic kidney disease / nephropathy, 150–53, *152*, *154*

diabetic muscle infarction, 181

diabetic retinopathy, 7, 112–15, *114*

diagnosis: ankle brachial index for, 169–70; of celiac disease, 144; of Charcot joint disease, 175; of congestive heart failure, 128; of cystic fibrosis–related diabetes, 24; of dawn phenomenon, 32–33; of dementia, 109; of diabetes, 11, *17*; of gastroparesis, 142; of gestational diabetes, 208; of hearing loss, 119; of heart disease, 127; of hypogonadism, 203; of macular edema, 117; of maturity-onset diabetes of young, 22–23; of nonalcoholic fatty liver disease, 146; of osteoporosis, 183; of pancreatic cancer, 190; of pancreatitis, 149–50; of peripheral neuropathy, 163; of peripheral vascular disease, 136; of polycystic ovarian syndrome, 214; of prediabetes, 19–20; of stroke, 106–7; of thyroid disease, 123–24; of type 2 diabetes in children, 63. *See also* testing

dialysis, 152–53, 157–58

diastolic blood pressure, 129–30

diastolic heart failure, 128

diet: apps to track, 94; counting carbohydrates, 84, 85–87, 90; for cystic fibrosis–related diabetes, 25; gluten-free, 144–45; in hospital, 76–77; for older adults, 66; plate method of meal planning, *88*, 89; popular diets, 91–94; to prevent diabetes, 6–7, 14–15; for type 1 diabetes, 83–87; for type 2 diabetes, 87–89

Dietary Approaches to Stop Hypertension (DASH) diet, 92

dietitians, 84, 86, 88, 93, 99

digital sclerosis, 177–78

disabilities: diabetes self-management and, 80; strokes and, 108

discrimination in workplace, 55–56

distal pancreatectomy, *26*

diuretics, 128, 276–77

DKA (diabetic ketoacidosis), *17*, 35–37, 238–39

domperidone, 143
dopamine agonists, *313*
DPP-4 inhibitors, 150, 221, 230, *231*, 232–33, *313*
driving, 53–55
drugs. *See* medications
dry skin, 179
dual-energy x-ray absorptiometry (DXA) scan, 183, 185
dulaglutide (Trulicity), 221, 233, *313*
duloxetine (Cymbalta), 164
dumping syndrome, 104
Dupuytren contracture, 182
dyslipidemia: managing, 131–33; medications for, 277–87; obesity and, 99

ears: hearing loss, 118–19; outer ear infections, 197–98
edema, 128
educational resources, 82
electrocardiograms (EKGs or ECGs), 127
emergencies: glucagon kits for, 41, 44; hyperglycemic, 35–39; preparation for, 53–54, 81
emotional care, 80
empagliflozin (Jardiance), 221, 238, *313*
employment and discrimination, 55–56
endocrinologists, 27, 129
endoscopy, 142
end-stage kidney disease, 152–53, 157–58
environment, as risk factor, 12
erectile dysfunction, 168, 199, 200–202
eruptive xanthomatosis, 179
erythromycin, 143
erythropoietin, 191
esophageal scintigraphy, 166
estrogen supplements, 210
ethnicity: health disparity and, 70–71; as risk factor, 13; type 2 diabetes and, 5
exenatide (Byetta or Bydureon), 221, 233, *313*
exercise, 14, 45, 66, 95–98, *96*
eyes: cataracts, 115–16; diabetic retinop-
athy, 7, 112–15, *114*; exams of, 45, 206; macular edema, 116–17
ezetimibe (Zetia), 279–80

family history, as risk factor, 13, *16*
fasting, religious, 73–74
fasting blood glucose, 11, 18
fenugreek, 265
fertility, 210
fiber, dietary, 85
fibric acid derivatives, 279, 283–84
fingers, pricking, 81, 293
Finnish diabetes prevention study, 6–7
fish oils, 281–83
flexor tenosynovitis, 182
food logs, 94
foot infections, 197
foot ulcers, 163, 168, 171–73, 178
Fortamet. *See* metformin
frozen shoulder, 182

gabapentin (Neurontin), 164
gadolinium, 155
gamma-blutamyl transpeptidase enzyme, 148
gastric emptying study, 166
gastric pacemaker, 143
gastroenterologists, 166–67
gastrointestinal tract, nerve damage in, 166–67
gastroparesis, 141–43, 166
genitals, infections of, 196
gestational diabetes, 1, 14, 207–9, 261
ginseng, 265
glimepiride (Amaryl), 221, 241, *312*
glipizide (Glucotrol), 221, 241, *312*
global burden of diabetes, 4–6
glomerular filtration rate (GFR), 151–52, *152*, 155
GLP-1 hormone, 232
GLP-1 receptor agonists: overview of, 233, *234*, 235–36, *313*, *314*; pancreatitis and, 150; for type 2 diabetes, 221; use with insulin, 250

glucagon, 149, 247, 249

glucagon injections, 41

glucocorticoid therapies, 28

Glucophage. *See* metformin

glucose: elevations in, 1–2, 32–33; optimal targets for, 7–9; self-monitoring of, 30–32, 45, 50, 217; testing level of, 11–12, 18–19

glucose meters, 30–31, *31*, 80, 291–93, *292*

glucose monitors, continuous (CGMs), 293–96, *294*, 309

glucose trend, 294

glutamic acid decarboxylase, 194, 195

gluten, sensitivity to, 143–45

glyburide (DiaBeta, Micronase, Glynase), 221, 241, *312*

glycemic index, 93

glycosylated hemoglobin, 33

granuloma annulare, 178

growth hormone, 32

gymnema, 265

hands, pain or stiffness in, 181–82

health care providers, use of term, x

health disparities, 70–71

hearing loss, 118–19

heart, nerve damage to, 167

heart disease. *See* cardiovascular disease

hemodialysis, 152–53, 157–58

hemoglobin, 192

hemoglobin A1C test, 12, 19, 33–35, *34*

hemorrhages in eyes, 113, *114*

hemorrhagic strokes, 105

hepatitis B vaccines, 49

heroin use, 57

high blood pressure. *See* hypertension

home blood glucose testing, 30–32, 45, 50. *See also* glucose meters

hormone replacement therapy, 212

hospital stays: diabetes care during, 74–78, *76*; glucose goals during, 9, 10

human immunodeficiency virus (HIV), 68–70

human leukocyte antigen (HLA) genes, 13

hyperglycemic emergencies: diabetic keto-acidosis, 35–37; hyperosmolar hypergly-cemia syndrome, *17*, 37–39

hyperosmolar hyperglycemia syndrome (HHS), *17*, 37–39

hypertension: ACE inhibitors for, 156, 269, *270*, 271–72, 273; ARBs for, 156, 269, 271, 272–73; beta-blockers for, 273–75; calcium channel blockers for, 275–76; control and prevention of, 130–31; diuretics for, 276–77; measurement of, 129–30; medications for, 128–29, 130–31; risk factors for, 130

hyperthyroidism, 122–23

hypoglycemia: after meals, 41–43, 104; bo-lus insulins and, 256; overnight, 43–44; prevention and treatment of, 39–41; risk of, *17*; tight control of glucose levels and, 7

hypoglycemia unawareness, 39

hypogonadism, 202–3

hypothyroidism, 122

immune-modulating therapies, 7

immune system, 193–94

impaired fasting glucose, 18

impaired glucose tolerance, 18

incretin mimetics, 233, *234*, 235–36

incretins, 2

infectious diseases, 196–98

influenza, 48–49, 197

inhaled insulin (Afrezza), 216, 217, 257–59, *258*, *311*

injections: common sites for, 219, *219*; drawing up insulin for, 81, 217; perform-ing, 216; site reactions, 176–77; site rotation, 256, 261, 263; switching from insulin pumps to, 77

insulin: basal, 250, *251*, 252–54, *253*, *311*; bolus, 254–57, *256*, *311*; for cystic fibrosis–related diabetes, 24; definition of, 1; inhaled, 216, 217, 257–59, *258*; menstrual cycle and, 213; pancreas in production of, 25, 149;

lixisenatide (Adlyxin), 221, 233, *313*

long-acting insulins. *See* basal (intermediate- and long-acting) insulins

lorcaserin (Belviq), 102

low blood glucose. *See* hypoglycemia

lung function and inhaled insulin, 258

macroalbuminuria, 151, 156

macular edema, 116–17

malignant otitis externa, 198

mantras, 266

marijuana use, 57

maturity-onset diabetes of the young (MODY), 22–23

meals, hypoglycemia after, 41–43, 104

medical alert bracelets, 40–41

medications: currently available, *311–14*; overview of, 216–24. *See also specific medications*

meditation and stress reduction, 266–68

Mediterranean Diet, 93

meglitinides, 221, 239, *240*, 241–42, *312*

menopause, 211–12

menorrhagia, 213

menstrual cycle, 212–13

metabolic syndrome, 133–34

metformin (Glucophage): action of, *226*; for children, 64; dosage and regimen for, 227; heart failure, lactic acidosis, and, 129; overview of, 225, 227–28; for PCOS, 215; for prediabetes, 20; for type 2 diabetes, 220

metoclopramide (Reglan), 142–43

microalbuminuria, 151, 156

microaneurysms, 113, *114*

miglitol (Glyset), 221, 228, *313*

mindfulness-based cognitive therapy, 267

mindfulness-based stress reduction, 267, *267*

mixed meal test, 42

MODY (maturity-onset diabetes of the young), 22–23

monitoring blood glucose. *See* continuous glucose monitors; glucose meters;

hemoglobin A1C test; self-monitoring of blood glucose

mouth, and tooth and gum disease, 119–21

mucormycosis, 198

musculoskeletal diseases, 180–83

myocardial infarctions (heart attacks), 124, *126*, 126–27

naltrexone/buproprion (Contrave), 102

nateglinide (Starlix), 221, 241, *312*

natural disasters, preparation for, 59–61

natural sweeteners, 90

necrobiosis lipodica diabeticorum, 178

nerve conduction study, 163

nervous system: autonomic neuropathy, 166–68; peripheral neuropathy, *162*, *162*, 162–65, *165*

neurodegenerative diseases, 108–10

neurologists, 165

niacin, 280–81

nocturnal hypoglycemia, 43–44

nonalcoholic fatty liver disease, 145–47

nonalcoholic steatohepatitis, 145

non-insulin injectable therapy. *See* GLP-1 receptor agonists

nonproliferative retinopathy, 112–13

Normoglycemia in Intensive Care Evaluation study, 9

NPH insulin (Humulin N, Novolin N), *218*, 250, *253*, *311*

Nutrisystem diet, 94

obesity: in children, 62, 64–65; managing, 99; medications for, 102; obstructive sleep apnea and, 138–39; surgery for, 102, 103–4

obstructive sleep apnea, 137–39, *140*

OGTT (oral glucose tolerance test), 11–12, 18–19

older adults, 65–68, *67*

oligomenorrhea, 213

omega-3 fatty acids, 281–83

optimal blood glucose targets, 7–9

oral combination pills, *314*

oral glucose tolerance test (OGTT), 11–12, 18–19

organ systems, 2, 3. *See also specific organs*

organ transplants: kidneys, 157, 158–60; pancreas and islet, 305, *306*, 307–8; pros and cons of, 307–8; steroid drugs and, 28

orlistat (Alli, Xenical), 102

orthostatic hypotension, 167

ospemifene (Osphena), 210

osteoarthritis, 180

osteopenia, 183

osteoporosis, 183–87, 211

overnight hypoglycemia, 43–44

over-the-counter medication, 50–51

pain of peripheral neuropathy, 164–65

pancreas: artificial, 308–10; cystic fibrosis and, 23, 24; function of, 1, 149, 305; impairment of, 2; transplantation of, 305, *306*, 307–8

pancreatic cancer, 189–90

pancreatic enzyme replacement, 27

pancreatic islets, 24, 25

pancreaticoduodenectomy (Whipple), *26*

pancreatic surgery, diabetes after, 25–28, *26*

pancreatitis: DPP-4 inhibitors and, 233; GLP-1 receptor agonists and, 236; overview of, 149–50; triglycerides and, 284

PAP (positive airway pressure), 139, *140*

partial pancreatectomy, *26*

PCOS (polycystic ovarian syndrome), 214–15

PCSK9 inhibitors, 286–87

PDE5 inhibitors, 200

pens, prefilled with insulin, 60, 80, 216, *217*, 252, 255

periodontal disease, 119–21

peripheral artery disease, 134–37

peripheral neuropathy, 162–65, *165*

peritoneal dialysis, 153, 158

perseverance, 80

phentermine/topiramate ER (Qsymia), 102

physical activity, 95–98. *See also* exercise

pioglitazone (Actos), 146–47, 221, 242, *313*

plaque in arteries, 124, *125, 136*

plate method of meal planning, *88, 89*

pneumonia, 49, 197

polycystic ovarian syndrome (PCOS), 214–15

positive airway pressure (PAP), 139, *140*

postpancreatectomy diabetes, 25–28, *26*

pramlintide (Symlin), 221, 249, *313*

prandial hypoglycemia, 41–43

prediabetes: defined, 4; lifestyle changes for, 14–15, 19–20; number of persons with, 5; in older adults, 65; testing for, 18–19

preeclampsia, 207

pregabalin (Lyrica), 164

pregnancy: ACE inhibitors in, 271; ARBs in, 273; aspirin in, 290; bolus insulins in, 256; gestational diabetes in, 1, 14, 207–9, 261; insulin secretagogues in, 242; metformin in, 228; overview of, 204–7; statins in, 279

premixed insulin preparations, 259–62, *260, 312*

prevention: of cancer, 189; of cardio-vascular disease, 287–90; of diabetes, 6–7, 9, 14–15, 19–20, 65; of diabetic retinopathy, 113, 115; of foot ulcers, 172; of hypertension, 130–31; of hypoglycemia, 40–41; of kidney damage, 7, 9; of osteoporosis, 184; routine preventive measures, 45, *46–47, 47*; of strokes, 107–8; of type 2 diabetes in children, 64

pricking fingers, 81, 293

Pritikin Weight Loss Breakthrough, 92

proliferative retinopathy, 113

proteinuria, 151

race and health disparities, 70–71

Ramadan fast, 73–74

random blood glucose, 11

rapid-acting insulins. *See* bolus insulins; inhaled insulin

reactive hypoglycemia, 41–43

regular insulin (Novolin R, Humulin R), *218, 255, 256, 311*

repaglinide (Prandin), 221, 241, *312*

research studies in diabetes care, 6–10

resistance training, 95–96, *96*

respiratory or lung infections, 197

retina, 112. *See also* diabetic retinopathy

risk factors: for amputation, 169, 171; for anemia, 192; for cancer, 187–88; for dawn phenomenon, 32; for diabetic ketoacidosis, 36; for foot ulcers, 172–73; for gestational diabetes, 207; for heart disease, 8, 109, 124, 126; for hyperosmolar hyperglycemia syndrome, 37–38; for hypertension, 130; for hypoglycemia, 17; for liver disease, 145–46; for nocturnal hypoglycemia, 43; overview of, *16*; for problems during fasting, 73–74; for steroid-induced diabetes, 28; for type 1 diabetes, 12–13; for type 2 diabetes, 13–15; for vitamin D deficiency, *186*

rosiglitazone (Avandia), 221, 242, *313*

Roux-en-Y gastric bypass, 104

saxagliptin (Onglyza), 221, 232, *313*

scleredema, 179

secretagogues, 239, *240*, 241–42

selective serotonin reuptake inhibitors (SSRIs), 111

self-monitoring of blood glucose, 30–32, 45, 50, 217. *See also* glucose meters

semaglutide (Ozempic), 221, 235, *313*

sensorineural hearing loss, 118–19

sepsis, 178

serotonin and norepinephrine reuptake inhibitors (SNRIs), 111

serving sizes, 86

sexual difficulties: of men, 168, 199–204; of women, 209–10

SGLT2 inhibitors, 221, 236, 237, *238*, 238–39, *313*

shin spots, 179

shoes, importance of, 172

short-acting insulins. *See* bolus insulins

shoulder dystocia, 206

shoulders, pain or stiffness in, 182–83

sick days, 49–51

silent heart attacks, 126–27

simple carbohydrates, 85

sinus infections, 198

sitagliptin (Januvia), 221, 232, *313*

skin conditions and infections, 176–80, 197

sleep and obstructive sleep apnea, 137–39, *140*

smoking, 57, 108, 258

SNRIs (serotonin and norepinephrine reuptake inhibitors), 111

social support, 51–53, 81, 97

South Beach Diet, 92

spironolactone, 215, 276

SSRIs (selective serotonin reuptake inhibitors), 111

statin medications, 108, 132, 277–79

steroid-induced diabetes, 28–29

stiff hand syndrome, 181

stiff person disease, 180–81

"stocking-glove" location of pain, *162*

strokes, 105–8, *107*

substance use, 56, *57*, 58–59

sucrose, 90

sugar, 85, 89

sugar alcohols, 90

sugar substitutes, 90

sulfonylureas, 221, 239, *240*, 241–42, *312*

support groups, 81

surgery for weight loss, 102, 103–4

surgical menopause, 211

sweating and nerve damage, 168

symptoms: of anemia, 192–93; of autonomic nerve damage, 166, 167; of cardiovascular disease, 97; of cataracts, 116; of celiac disease, 144;

symptoms (*cont.*)
of depression, 110–11; of diabetes, *16*; of diabetic ketoacidosis, 36–37; of gastroparesis, 142; of hearing loss, 119; of heart attack, *126*, 126–27; of hyperosmolar hyperglycemia syndrome, 38; of hypoglycemia, 39, *40*; of kidney disease, 155; of liver disease, 147–48; of low testosterone, 202–3; of nocturnal hypoglycemia, 43–44; of obstructive sleep apnea, 139; of pancreatic cancer, 190; of pancreatitis, 149; of periodontal disease, 121; of peripheral vascular disease, 134–35; of polycystic ovarian syndrome, 214; of strokes, 105–6; of thyroid disease, 122–23
syringes, 216, *217*, 252, *254*, 255, 263
systolic blood pressure, 129
systolic heart failure, 127–28

talk therapy for depression, 111
tardive dyskinesia, 143
testing: for albuminuria, 156–57; for autoantibodies, 193–96; for diabetes, 11–12; hemoglobin A1C test, 33–35, *34*; home blood glucose test, 30–32, 45, 50; for kidney function, 153, 155; for liver disease, 147–48; for prediabetes, 18–20; for reactive hypoglycemia, 42; for vitamin D deficiency, 185–87. *See also* glucose meters
testosterone, 201, 202–4
test strips with glucose meters, 31, *292*, 292–93
Therapeutic Lifestyle Changes diet, 92
thiazolidinediones, 129, 221, 242, *243*, 244, 313
thrombectomy, 107
thyroid disease, 122–24
tissue plasminogen activator (tPA), 106
tooth and gum disease, 119–21
total pancreatectomy, 26
transcendental meditation, 266
trans fats, 89

transplantation: of kidneys, 157, 158–60; of pancreas and islets, 305, *306*, 307–8
treatment: of anemia, 193; of cataracts, 116; of celiac disease, 144–45; of Charcot joint disease, 175; cost of, 5; of cystic fibrosis–related diabetes, 24; of dawn phenomenon, 33; of dementia, 109; of depression, 111–12; of diabetes, 4, *17*, *311–14*; of diabetic ketoacidosis, 37; of erectile dysfunction, 201–2; of gastroparesis, 142–43; of gestational diabetes, 208–9; of hearing loss, 119; of high cholesterol, 132; of hyperosmolar hyperglycemia syndrome, 38–39; of hypogonadism, 203–4; of kidney disease, 157–58; of LADA, 21–22; of macular edema, 117; of maturity-onset diabetes of the young, 23; of menopausal symptoms, 212; of metabolic syndrome, 134; of nocturnal hypoglycemia, 44; of nonalcoholic fatty liver disease, 146–47; of obstructive sleep apnea, 139, *140*; for older adults, 67–68; of osteoporosis, 184–85; of pain of peripheral neuropathy, 164–65; of pancreatitis, 150; of periodontal disease, 121; of peripheral vascular disease, 137; of polycystic ovarian syndrome, 215; postpancreatectomy diabetes, 27; of reactive hypoglycemia, 42–43; of retinopathy, 115; of steroid-induced diabetes, 29; of vitamin D deficiency, 187. *See also* complementary and alternative treatments; lifestyle changes; medications
tuberculosis, 197
type 1 diabetes: autoantibody testing and, 193–96; insulin treatment for, 216–17, *217, 218,* 219; LADA, 20–22; nutrition for, 83–87; overview of, 1; pancreas in, 2; prevention of, 9; risk factors for, 12–13; treatment of, 4, 247–62, *311*; type 2 diabetes compared to, 15, *15–17,* 18
type 2 diabetes: in children, 62–65; ethnicity and, 5; incretins and, 2; insulin treatment for, 221, 222–24; LADA com-

pared to, 21; non-insulin treatment for, 220–22; nutrition for, 87–89; overview of, 1; risk factors for, 13–15; treatment of, 4, *311–14*; type 1 diabetes compared to, 15, *15–17*, 18. *See also* prediabetes

U-500 regular concentrated insulin, 262–63
UK Prospective Diabetes Study, 8
uremia, 157
urinary incontinence, 160–61
urinary tract infections, 167–68, 196
urine albumin to creatinine ratio, 155

vaccinations, 45, 48–49
vanadium, 265
velvety skin, 179
Veterans Affairs Diabetes Trial, 9
vials for insulin, 216, 217, 252, 254, 255, 263
vipassana, 267–68
virus exposure, as risk factor, 12–13

vision loss, 7, 9. *See also* diabetic retinopathy; eyes
vitamin D, 264

weight loss: benefits of, 91, 99; PCOS and, 215; programs for, 91–94; surgery for, 102, 103–4; type 2 diabetes and, 87
Weight Watchers, 93–94
women's health: menopause, 211–12; menstrual cycle, 212–13; polycystic ovarian syndrome, 214–15; sexual difficulties, 209–10. *See also* pregnancy
wound healing, 173–74

yeast infections, 178, 196
yellow nails, 179
yoga poses, 267

zinc transporter autoantibodies (ZnT8), 194, 195
Zone Diet, 93
zygomycete, 178

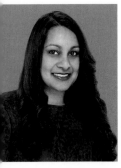

RITA R. KALYANI, MD, MHS, is an associate professor of medicine in the Division of Endocrinology, Diabetes, and Metabolism at the Johns Hopkins University School of Medicine. She is the past chair of the American Diabetes Association's Professional Practice Committee, which establishes internationally recognized clinical practice guidelines, including the *Standards of Medical Care in Diabetes*, that are used by health care providers around the world. A graduate of Harvard College, she completed her medical school, residency, and endocrinology and metabolism fellowship at the Johns Hopkins University School of Medicine and is board-certified in endocrinology and metabolism.

MARK D. CORRIERE, MD, is an adjunct assistant professor of medicine in the Division of Endocrinology, Diabetes, and Metabolism at the Johns Hopkins

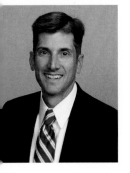

University School of Medicine. He attended medical school at Washington University and completed his internal medicine residency at the National Naval Medical Center in Bethesda, Maryland. He proudly served as a physician in the U.S. Navy for over a decade. He completed his endocrinology and metabolism fellowship at the Johns Hopkins University School of Medicine and is a board-certified clinical endocrinologist at Maryland Endocrine.

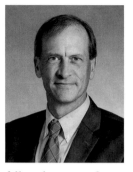 THOMAS W. DONNER, MD, is an associate profes
sor of medicine in the Division of Endocrinology, Di
abetes, and Metabolism at the Johns Hopkins Univer
sity School of Medicine. He holds the Jules and Joan
Edlow Endowed Professorship in Diabetes and is di
rector of the Johns Hopkins Comprehensive Diabete
Center. He received his medical degree from the Uni
versity of Virginia School of Medicine and completed
his internal medicine residency, chief residency, and
fellowship in endocrinology and metabolism at the University of Maryland
School of Medicine. He is board-certified in endocrinology and metabolism.

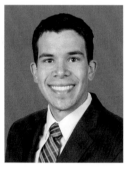 MICHAEL W. QUARTUCCIO, MD, is an adjunct as
sistant professor of medicine in the Division of En
docrinology, Diabetes, and Metabolism at the Johns
Hopkins University School of Medicine. He attend
ed medical school at Jefferson Medical College and
completed his internal medicine residency and chief
residency at the University of Maryland Medical Cen
ter. He completed his endocrinology and metabolism
fellowship at the Johns Hopkins University School of
Medicine and is a board-certified clinical endocrinologist in the Rochester Re
gional Health System.

**Endnotes, Index, Illustrations Credits, About the Authors
to come**